YOUR BRAIN ON CUBS

YOUR BRAIN ON CUBS

Inside the Heads of Players and Fans

EDITED BY DAN GORDON

DANA
PRESS

New York • Washington, D.C.

Copyright 2008, all rights reserved
Published by Dana Press
New York/Washington, D.C.

The Dana Foundation
745 Fifth Avenue, Suite 900
New York, NY 10151
900 15th Street NW
Washington, DC 20005
DANA is a federally registered trademark.
www.dana.org

ISBN-13: 978-1-932594-28-7
Library of Congress Cataloging-in-Publication Data
Your brain on Cubs : inside the heads of players and fans /
edited by Dan Gordon.
p. cm.
ISBN-13: 978-1-932594-28-7
1. Chicago Cubs (Baseball team)   2. Baseball fans—
Psychology.   3. Baseball players—Psychology.
I. Gordon, Dan.
GV875.C6Y68 2008
796.357'640977311—dc22
2007048474

Cover Design by Tobias' Outerwear for Books

CONTENTS

PREFACE

When I'm not editing books and periodicals about the brain, I'm a violinist by avocation. On September 30, 2003, I attended my rehearsal with the Washington Conservatory Orchestra and missed seeing the Cubs defeat the Atlanta Braves in the first game of that year's National League Division Series. The Cubs went on to win that series, three games to one.

Two weeks later, a night on which a Cubs victory would send the team to the World Series for the first time in 58 years, I made the same choice: to attend rehearsal and then hope to catch the last two innings of the ball game. No reason, I thought, to press my luck by skipping rehearsal this time; after all, the strategy had worked two weeks prior. I wouldn't want to jinx them.

I somehow stayed focused at rehearsal, and my strategy seemed to be working again: afterward, as I drove to the Irish pub where my friends were watching the game, I listened on the radio as the Cubs took a 3–0 lead into the late innings. I panicked briefly when I couldn't find a parking space, afraid that I wouldn't be watching when the Cubs sealed the deal.

But the game wasn't over when I raced into the bar. In fact, there was one out in the top of the 8th inning, with the Florida Marlins up to bat. The Cubs were five outs away from the Series.

Not sixty seconds after I started watching, Luis Castillo of the Marlins hit a pop foul into the front row in left field. The Cubs' left fielder might have caught the ball for the inning's second out, but a fan made a play on it instead. From there the inning and the series unraveled for the Cubs, along with our dreams of a World Series appearance and victory.

Fans blamed the man who had reached for the foul ball— and there's more on him later in this book. But for a while, I felt as though I should have pretended there was no game at all—as though that would have allowed my team to cruise to victory. Clearly I'd changed their fortunes by showing up to watch.

Such is the life of a Cubs fan: As if a curse involving a billy goat weren't enough, even the most rational among us are prone to believing that we somehow contributed to the team's failures.

It was not until the following season, on a sun-soaked June afternoon at Wrigley Field, that I began to realize that the very existence of such a thing as sports fandom grows out of the way the brain works. What, in my brain, made me loyal and hopeful enough to come back despite disappointment that still seemed fresh? Why is Wrigley Field considered by so many people to be beautiful, relative to other ballparks? What was responsible for the rush I felt when the Cubs recorded the last out in what had become a dominating, 6–1 victory?

Other questions popped up over time: What part of the ballplayer's brain makes him able to hit a pitch traveling at perhaps ninety-five miles per hour, coming from less than sixty feet away? How does a ballplayer develop superlative skill at a position and at the plate?

Admittedly, it took longer for me to consider my brain's role in permitting my belief that I had jinxed the team on that October night. We do not like to admit our own irrationality, even if we share it with legions of fans who believe their team is cursed.

Perhaps, one day, that same superstition will allow us to believe that we contributed to our team's triumph. But we Cubs fans know better than to hope for such a day.

In fact, when I first drafted this preface, the Cubs were days away from their first playoff series since 2003. I considered making plans for how this book would have to change should they go on to make the World Series, perhaps even win it. But I didn't want to jinx them.

It didn't matter. The Cubs lost the division series to the Arizona Diamondbacks in startlingly quick fashion. I returned to orchestra rehearsal without conflict, without superstition—and frankly without the heartache of 2003. A cynic could argue that at least the Cubs had the decency to spare us from hope this time.

But hope we will—with all our hearts, and with a great deal of our brains. There's always next year.

Dan Gordon
November 2007

- 1 -

THE DEPTHS OF LOYALTY
Exploring the Brain of a Die-hard Fan

JORDAN GRAFMAN, PH.D.

INTRODUCTION

I confess that I am a lifelong Cubs fan and this chapter will present a biased, personal view. If being a fan of a football team is like having an affair (short seasons and long drives), being a baseball fan is like being in a marriage (long seasons, slower pace, and a focus on details).

My first memories of the Cubs go back to the mid- to late 1950s, when I would come home from Armstrong Elementary School in Rogers Park in Chicago and find my dad sitting in the living room, watching the Cubs on WGN-TV. Despite having a few stars such as Ernie Banks, the Cubs of that era were dull compared to the South Side "go-go" Chicago White Sox (endorsed by Mayor Richard J. Daley), who won the American League pennant in 1959. Instead, the Cubs were beset by players such as the homerless Elvin Tappe and empty grandstand seats in April signaling that the cold

Canadian winds that blew hard through the ballpark could routinely influence not only the outcome of games at Wrigley but also the fans' level of support. As the Cubs play-by-play announcer of the 1950s and early 1960s, Jack Brickhouse, used to say between the rare "Hey-Heys"—his signature home run call—"Any team can have a bad century."

In fact, the Chicago Cubs played good baseball throughout the first half of the twentieth century following the Tinker to Evers to Chance era of the early 1900s, but for nearly 100 years, they have not won the baseball world championship. At one point in the late 1930s, the team even hired a sports psychologist to try to determine how to improve the team's performance. A fan of the Cubs must love the team with an almost religious fervor, given their tumultuous ups and downs.

They have had seasons where they looked like they could compete in and win the World Series. In 1969, I was in Shea Stadium in September courtesy of my Long Island cousin, Jeff, who took me to see the Mets play the Cubs in what would be for me the ultimate loss. We had to leave the game early to beat the traffic back out to Long Island and just after we left, the Mets scored a run to take the lead, and eventually the victory, from the Cubs. What I most remember from that day is the very long drive back to Long Island, with Jeff's monologue on the greatness of the '69 Mets and New York teams in general and laughing about what indeed ended up being the Cubs' slow, tortuous slide into infamy that year.

Having spent the first twenty years of my life in Chicago, I was indoctrinated to the idea that actions speak louder than words and that we were the "City of Broad Shoulders." So I often wondered why I remained a Cubs fan despite the singularity of their failures over the years. Was my optimism simply a form of magical thinking, a form of fantasy on the borderline between reality and dreams? Enjoying a baseball game was supposed to be a recreational activity, a chance to forget about life and to simply follow the play on the field. I often took the short ride on the B train from where I lived to get to Addison and the "friendly confines" of Wrigley Field, and at least sitting in the bleachers with no protection from the sun kept you warm on a spring day when you were supposed to be at school. But I am not sure that I explicitly understood the paradox of rooting for a team that was destined to frustrate both their fans and the idea of watching baseball as an escape from life's problems. Perhaps, as a cognitive neuroscientist, I can now try to rationalize this madness.

A fan's dedication to a chronically losing baseball team involves a number of social-cognitive processes that allow him to accept his fate, along with other aesthetic appreciations related to the field of play. In the case of a losing team, a fan has to be prepared to delay gratification for years, decades, and occasionally a century (the latter case involves handing down the delayed gratification to subsequent generations of family fans, entrusting them to appreciate the long road to the ultimate victory). A fan also must make an effort to reduce an intrinsic motivation to analyze management's apparent lack of interest in the team or a player's self-interest that seems to overshadow the coherence and success of the team. Despite these factors, and even if we reduce their impact on our hopes for the team, how do we maintain our conviction that the team will one day be victorious?

There is some evidence that being in the majority (everyone loves a winner) reduces reflective thinking, whereas being in the minority (rooting for a loser) increases reflection. Perhaps that reflection is rewarding in itself and helps motivate fans to root for a losing team (in that sense it is the chase that is important rather than the ultimate victory). What about the bonding between people that occurs when fans root for a perennial loser? Is any city better prepared to do this than Chicago, a working person's city? Even being in a losing "in group" may enhance self-esteem and strengthen group identity and, in the end, such a group identity may influence the individual person's identity. The fun part for me, as a cognitive neuroscientist, is that all these social processes are mediated by specific brain regions and therefore it is exciting to speculate on what it is that keeps us rooting for a team so prone to disappointing us. This can be revealing for fans of all teams and all sports—and for those (e.g., sports widows) who try to understand us.

DELAYING GRATIFICATION

As every Cubs fan knows, there are at least two goals in going to watch a baseball game at beautiful Wrigley Field. One is short-term and can be attained on the same day as the game being played, and that is simply enjoying being in a ballpark that is entrenched in a city neighborhood with friends, hopefully seeing both a well-played game and a victory for Chicago. The other goal is long-term and not necessarily in conflict with the short-term goal: winning the world championship. It has been almost half a century since I was photographed with my Cubs hat on in Chicago at the end of another dismal season, one that Cubs shortstop Ernie Banks's exceptional play could not remedy!

So how do we Cubs fans (and fans of other losing fran-

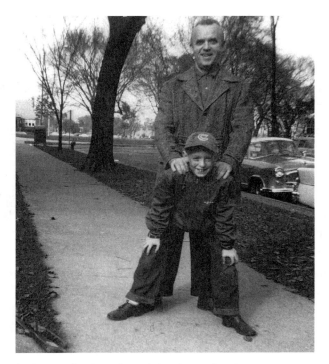

A photograph taken of my dad and me when I was seven years old, following a typically mediocre Cubs baseball season. Note the counterfactual happiness in my face.

chises—here's looking at you, Houston) deal with delaying the ultimate gratification that is winning the World Series? One obvious solution is to develop explicit strategies for coping with an unmet long-term goal, including rationalizations about the eventual joy, the path to winning being as important as the ultimate victory, the fun of the day, and the importance of the unifying experience of the crowd even during a loss. These go hand-in-hand with a reverse psychology that enshrines the team with a sort of loser's admiration. It has worked for me.

TOLERATING WEAKNESS—OR, ACCEPTING THE CURRENT CONDITION SO THAT UNDESIRABLE EVIDENCE IS NOT IGNORED

So even if celebrating a World Series victory is delayed, how can fans accept the current climate and keep from becoming morose without ignoring evidence such as a weak starting rotation, slumping batters, or little postseason experience? This clearly requires distancing oneself personally from the ups and downs of the team while still maintaining enthusiasm, interest, and loyalty. The distancing must be done in a way that keeps the team's poor performance from affecting personal identity and lessening personal involvement (in essence, this is like going along with the ups and downs of a long-term marriage). We humans do this often, and our ability to explicitly place such an activity in the proper context of our life is important to keeping it up.

KEEPING YOUR CONVICTIONS

In essence, reading about your team, hearing others' opinions that converge with and deviate from your own, and attending games in the presence of other fans all provide a cognitive narrative that enables you to keep your convictions positive. This kind of narrative can also be a "perennial loser" type of narrative that allows you to appear to others as an appealing underdog. Picking out virtues where you can find them, including the joy of watching a game of baseball at Wrigley Field, enables a fan to construct an adaptive narrative of hope that maintains convictions in the presence of undermining evidence—particularly when the narrative is shared among a large cadre of fans.

ARE CUBS FANS A MAJORITY OR MINORITY?

While sports fans tend to be loyal to a local team, everyone loves a winner. A fan living in the Washington, D.C., area might root for the New York Yankees rather than the Washington Nationals or Baltimore Orioles independent of whether he grew up in New York City because perennial winners tend to attract large numbers of fans, maybe a majority of fans of the sport across the country. Being in a majority group has numerous advantages both psychologically and politically, including the perception that it means you made a correct decision. Being a fan of a perennially losing team has little general advantage. It takes persistence and a willingness to work hard at being a fan after deciding to root for a loser. On the bright side, the scientific literature suggests that fans of losing teams turn out to be better decision-makers and deal better with divergent thought, as opposed to the unreflective fans of winning teams such as those from New York City. Since the fans of losing teams must have some cognitive dissonance between their choice of team and the evidence that it is not doing well, they must have to deliberate longer, and be more creative, to come up with a rationale for their choice of team. This effort can lead these fans to refine their decision-making and inferential reasoning skills to a superior level that would not be required by fans of consistently winning teams.

HOW DO CUBS FANS AS A GROUP IDENTIFY WITH THE TEAM?

We are born with endowed human characteristics that enable us to develop individual and group identities. But some group identities are also acquired through experience. We are not born Cubs fans but it is possible to receive proper Cubs fan training quite early in life. Sitting in the stands at Wrigley Field or watching a game at a public venue such as a bar or among friends at an apartment allows a group to cohere by binding individual identities and enabling the Cubs fan identity to be rewarded and ranked among other pleasurable activities of daily life. The costs of being a Cubs fan—or a fan of any team, for that matter—usually arise when an individual is a minority among members of another group— such as when attending a road game at Busch Stadium, home of the archrival St. Louis Cardinals. But the costs are outweighed by the more frequent experience of being among Cubs fans. The acknowledgment by other fans that you are a member of their group is rewarding and supportive. This is not surprising given the history of the social benefit of all kinds of group identities: families, tribes, religions, political parties, even regional and nationalistic identities. Obviously, being a fan of the Chicago Cubs doesn't engage some of the more meaningful aspects of other forms of group identities, but in a Western culture that is designed to minimize some of the more oppressive aspects of group identities, identifying yourself as a fan of a sports team can provide a relatively safe identity as well as increase personal value (i.e., I must be an okay person if I am a member of a group that is large and has the same general interests as I do, even if I am not a fanatical member of that group).

A FAN'S SELF-ESTEEM

Self-esteem can affect our self-image and influence how we behave with others. Being a Cubs fan does allow the enhancement of self-esteem within a certain range. After all, the Cubs play at beautiful Wrigley Field, and being able to watch a game there is a privilege. When the team does play well, which has happened at times during the past century, rooting for the team is validated, as is the fan who chooses to root for the team.

There is another, smaller contribution to self-esteem that involves the identification of the team with the City of Chicago. Although Chicago's mayors during the past half century have been either overt fans of a lesser-known team from the South Side or at best presumably neutral, most fans who live in the geographical region in which the team plays also identify with the shared characteristics of the area. This team, after all, is the *Chicago* Cubs. It is possible to bend the identity of the team toward the city's most publicized characteristics (i.e., it works, it is the City of Broad Shoulders, it has been Democratic with a flavor of socialism and corruption, it is honest in that the citizens prefer to stab you in the chest rather than in the back, it has at least a façade of Midwest helpfulness, and it keeps a sense of humor about itself) and thereby broaden the entity with which the home fan identifies. That, in turn, allows an increase of self-esteem that comes with being part of an even larger group (people who live in the Chicago region). And yes, this potential improvement in self-esteem can even help people in their search for the meaning of life since we often find metaphors for life in sports activities, and the Cubs have given us many.

PERSISTENCE AND ADAPTIVITY OF SOCIAL AND PERSONAL IDENTITIES

There is sufficient evidence that people integrate their personal identities with their social identities. Being a sports fan may be one instance where this integration becomes rather transparent to the observer. People readily wear T-shirts, hats, and insignias that identify them with a certain social group, and by far the biggest sellers are for sports teams or individual athletes. While it is possible for the category of *Cubs fan* to imply certain characteristics that are independent of any individual Cubs fan, it is likely that people choose to be Cubs fans because of certain relevant characteristics of fandom that overlap with their own self-identity, some of which have been described above. The persistence of this allegiance and identification with the Cubs is in part dependent upon the team's near-mythical inability to reach and win the World Series.

But what if the hoped-for were to happen? What if the Cubs won the World Series? What if they won more than one championship over a short period of time? Certainly that would eliminate a certain amount of angst and might even precipitate an identity crisis and a reevaluation of what is important about being a Chicago Cubs fan. Can we look elsewhere to analyze the effect? How about the Boston Red Sox, who overcame their own "curse" and won the World Series in 2004 (and then won again in 2007)?

There is no obvious lesson from observing Red Sox fans after their team's World Series wins except perhaps for reports of a drop-off of intensity of feeling about the Red Sox subsequent to their championships. Would the nostalgia for the feeling of rooting for a loser diminish? Would a percentage of Cubs fans drop by the wayside as their long-term goal was fulfilled? Would they—could they—adapt to a new identity as a winner? The stereotypical arrogance of a northeasterner is not part of the personality of a Chicagoan, so perhaps the expectation of future championships would be modulated in a Chicagoan compared to, say, a New Yorker.

Could we adjust? I like to dream.

SUMMARY OF THE SOCIAL-COGNITIVE CONSEQUENCES OF BEING A FAN

The social psychology literature is a wonderful source of information on the personal consequences of engaging in social activities, including being a fan of a sports team. Thus, it should not be surprising that being a baseball fan results in a number of social-cognitive and related processes being activated in various combinations and at various times in keeping with changes in the immediate environment, interests, and, of course, the fortunes of the team. These social processes include becoming an expert in delaying gratification, being able to balance good and bad information, developing a conviction that is not disabling about a perennial loser, establishing an identity with a social group, bonding with that same social group, maintaining self-esteem, and developing both a social and personal identity that takes into account affection for and interest in the team.

While at first blush these processes may seem common to many social endeavors, what makes these social processes unique for Cubs fans is that they play out in the context of the longevity of the team's frustration and the importance of the team for their identity in the world. Interestingly enough, these same general social processes have begun to be explored in human cognitive neuroscience experiments that use functional neuroimaging to study healthy volunteers while they perform social tasks or to study patients with brain damage in regions known to be important for the storage and execution of social processes. The results of these experiments allow me to imagine how the brain of a Cubs fan might function under certain circumstances.

SOCIAL NEUROSCIENCE: THE BRAIN
OF A CUBS FAN

What are the brain areas that every fan uses to increase his knowledge about the team, convey his desires regarding the team's decisions, help to form his explicit and implicit identity, and modulate the moods that are influenced by the performance of the team? Of course, I use my entire brain when I think about the Cubs, but certain areas are likely to be more important for the social processes required for a Cubs fan. For the purpose of illustration of these key brain areas, I have adapted a figure from a recent review chapter my colleagues and I wrote about the neural representation of moral cognition (see figure 1). The issues and brain structures discussed in that chapter were broad enough to be applicable to the social issues that I believe are critical for being a loyal fan.

The figure depicts brain areas concerned with emotion, including structures such as the amygdala that are part of the limbic system; areas concerned with reward, including the ventral tegmentum and ventral striatum; areas concerned with bonding, including the subgenual cortex and septum; areas concerned with social knowledge, such as the ventromedial prefrontal cortex; and areas concerned with explicit and implicit knowledge about the self—also contained within the prefrontal cortex. All these brain areas are connected to each other, forming flexible systems of brain activation depending on how your team is doing in the standings, your non-sports interactions at a particular moment, and, of course, your other non-sports-related goals. To make it easier to understand how the brain responds when thinking about our team of choice, it helps to consider some of the more typical situations a Cubs

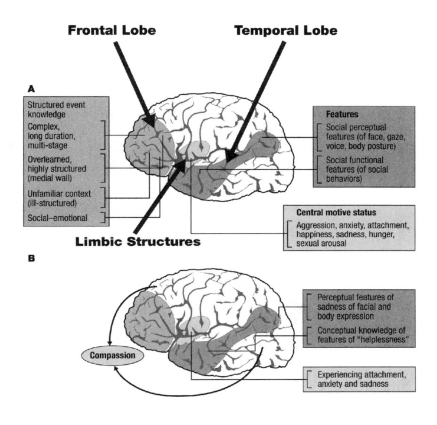

Figure 1. The brain-behavior framework that is relevant for a Cubs fan shows that the various behavioral states that Cubs fans experience emerge from the activation and binding of three main components: structured event knowledge (provided by context-dependent memory representations in subregions of the frontal lobes), social semantic and functional features (stored in the posterior and anterior sectors of the temporal cortex), and central motive or basic emotional states (such as aggressiveness, sadness, attachment, or joy, represented in brain-stem, limbic, and paralimbic regions). Courtesy of Jordan Grafman.

fan might find himself in and how brain activity corresponds to psychological states in those situations.

Given the complex situations and thinking that Cubs fans have had to engage in, it turns out that the frontal lobes are consistently activated in almost all circumstances involving a fan thinking about his team.

THE OVERALL HOPE FOR A WORLD SERIES CHAMPION ON THE NORTH SIDE

Though some might point to the past century as evidence that hoping for a championship requires losing one's mind, the hope in fact comes from a part of the brain called the prefrontal cortex. This brain region is known to be important for planning, reasoning, social cognition, knowledge about the behavior of others, establishing a context, and similar higher-level cognitive processes. The purpose of activation in this region would be to generate (obviously by analogy to other teams and situations) what the Cubs need to do to win the World Series, to retrieve knowledge about the fate of other teams that have won it, to inhibit the historical evidence related to the Cubs' failure to go all the way, and to temper any unrealistic assumptions about winning with hopeful longer-term goals—if the past is a guide, the goals must be very long-term indeed.

THE ENJOYMENT OF SITTING AT WRIGLEY FIELD WATCHING THE CUBS PLAY

Nostalgia about the intimacy of old baseball parks, social bonding with other fans watching or listening to the game, and encoding and predicting the sequence of events occurring on the day of the game (including aspects of the action itself) also activate the prefrontal cortex. However, more posterior brain regions concerned with visual, auditory, and even tactile perception and the emotion-centered limbic system become activated when you feel the wind in your hair coming from the north and west, view the beautiful green of the vines adorning the outfield walls, inhale the smell of a ballpark hot dog, look upon the natural turf of the outfield, and sense that your behavior is mirroring that of the fans around you and even the fans on the rooftops of the apartment buildings beyond the outfield bleachers. Your auditory cortex would take delight in hearing even the off-tune singing of "Take Me Out to the Ball Game" during the seventh-inning stretch. Your limbic system is also attuned to your mood as you follow the ups and downs of the Cubs' fortunes during the game, hopefully ending with a victory. In that instance, the brain's reward system, including the ventral brain stem and basal ganglia, would be pumping dopamine into your brain with a refinement that matches the experience of seeing the froth of a congratulatory beer at a neighborhood bar after the win. (The beer's effects in the brain involve the reward system described above, as well as the prefrontal cortex.)

SOCIAL BONDING

Sitting with friends at the game, hearing or discussing the game with the fans around you, or listening to it on a radio or watching it on TV allows for bonding with others. Such bonding activates the septum and the subgenual prefrontal cortex, which then release chemicals such as oxytocin that signal the degree of pleasure of the bonding. (For example, a mother's brain is pumping oxytocin as she bonds with her infant.) For some people, this bonding is powerful and brings a person back to the same situation—a particular baseball park, for example—many times in the future to experience the pleasure of this interpersonal bonding again.

WHO AM I?

The prefrontal cortex is also an essential brain region for mediating our notion of self. For example, watching a baseball team play may activate memories of playing baseball in our youth. Neuroscientists have identified so-called mirror neurons in our brain that are activated whether we engage in playing a sport *or* watch others play. This mirror neuron brain system spans frontal and posterior brain regions. It helps us integrate the enjoyment of playing the game with simple knowledge of the game and memories of our playing it in our youth. As Vittorio Gallese showed in a 2007 study, mirror neurons become activated when we watch a baseball team play.

Besides this implicit interplay between watching a sports team play and our own memories of who we were (and are), the love of a sports team is powerful enough for some people to influence their habits and schedules and motivate the way they form relationships with friends, relatives, spouses, and children. For the serious sports fan, this has obvious consequences: not everyone wants to devote a corner of the family room to a shrine for the team. In extraordinary circumstances, a sports team can galvanize a nation, giving the population something to identify with in a way little else could achieve.

For example, a few years ago I was in Greece, lecturing at a neuropsychology summer school. It so happened that the Greek national soccer team was competing for the European championship. Clearly an underdog, they won the championship that summer. The remarkable outpouring of happiness and emotion from the majority of Greeks, many of whom no doubt paid little attention to the team or the sport ordinarily, was particularly touching. Their country had won a major championship, and the celebrations lasted throughout the night. Touching though it was, thanks to my mirror neurons, watching the celebrations made the Cubs fan in me a bit wistful.

The Cubs will always remain a part of their fans' personal identities. This is symbolic—the overwhelming majority of fans have never met a player, nor do we consider them friends. We understand that they are businessmen, that different players represent the team at different times, under different owners whose business interests trump any sense of loyalty to the city. But we ignore these counterfactuals in order to lay our symbolism on the team, dress them up with our accumulated identities, and wait for the transcendent moment they win the big one and our identities become magically transformed.

PUTTING IT ALL TOGETHER

The social-cognitive and brain-research findings I have described are consistent in identifying both the kinds of social processes and the brain regions that underlie love not just of the Cubs, Wrigley Field, and the World Series chase, but of any team we root for as we dream of a championship. Although the content of Cubs fans' experiences is uniquely stored in our brains, the social processes under which that content operates, as well as the brain mechanisms we need to support those processes, are not unique to sports fandom. The same regions of the brain are activated by other parts of our identity concerned with work, family, and hobbies. The neural representations of the Cubs and these other parts of our lives overlap in the brain and include systems that we have for signifying emotional states, bonding in relationships, thinking about the past and the future, enjoying a sensual experience, and forming a sense of self.

Yet there are few threads in our life that follow us from childhood through adulthood, even to the edge of passing on. These threads allow us to retrieve a memory, a powerful memory from youth, and reexperience it as if it were yesterday, with all the primitive feelings a young boy or girl can have. I remember playing a pickup game of hardball at the local park in my neighborhood in Chicago in the early '60s. This particular game involved a team of mostly younger kids such as myself, still in elementary school, and a team of mostly older boys, some of whom had just entered high school. Amazingly, we were winning in the ninth inning. A ball was hit toward me. After a long run, and with an outstretched glove, I caught it, preserving the victory. My friends gathered round me and we hugged and laughed, and perhaps for a single moment we thought of ourselves as the Cubs of our dreams.

This is a powerful memory, one that far outweighs the objective triviality of that particular game and its overall importance in my life. No doubt that memory will remain with me for as long as I live. It is linked to the team that I began to follow in the days when my dad was alive and I joined him in the living room after school to watch the Cubs play, kept rooting for during the horror of the Mets' miracle season in 1969, and was still cheering the year manager Dusty Baker patted my wife's pregnant abdomen for luck in the middle of a season that began to deteriorate with an infamous foul ball. The memory lives on in my recent attempts to pass my love of the Cubs to my young sons. The depth of my loyalty to that team (and city) has far transcended the time I lived in Chicago and the years that have passed since my childhood.

As a cognitive neuroscientist I have been taught to study my subjects with tightly controlled experiments and stimuli so I can generalize my results to all kinds of people and situations. Although these kinds of experiments can be extremely important, they occasionally miss the sense of real-life knowledge and identification that comes with studying people in situations they are familiar with and enjoy. Yet there is an obvious link between the brain, social behavior, and being a baseball fan that I hope that I have conveyed.

As I write these words, Chicago is in first place in the Midwest Division of the National League, barely ahead of the Milwaukee Brewers. It makes me want to close my eyes and dream, with the deep hope etched in a loyal Cubs fan's brain, about the World Series.

DEVELOPING TALENT

Expertise and the Brain

SCOTT GRAFTON, M.D.

It's Thursday evening at the ballpark. Up in the bleachers, peanuts in hand, you have a fine view of both the mound and home plate. The game has been close, with plenty of hits and base stealing to keep you interested. Here comes your child up to bat. It is time for you, the parent, to face the music. Is your kid any good or not? All those sports camps, the coaching, the endless practice. Is any of it going to make your kid a star player? Your child likes to play and is happy with her teammates. But will her talent last more than a season?

Just as your mind wanders on this fundamental parenting question, your daughter uncorks a line drive over the shortstop. Making it to second base without a moment to spare, she recaptures your attention. Maybe all that practice does matter. Or perhaps, unlikely as it may appear at first, she is a one-in-a-million "natural," as if born exclusively for this sport, with practice simply tuning up a gift she already seems to have.

Every parent considers versions of these thoughts in one form or another: sports, violin lessons, art classes, dance, science camp. And if our children are not naturals in these skills, maybe the best to expect is that they are passionate in pursuing them. This tension between what kids are born with and what they gain from practice is at the core of understanding what it takes to become an expert. It is also at the center of understanding how neuroscientists approach the question of defining what the brain of an expert looks like and how it might function differently compared to the merely competent. A look at what makes expert ballplayers must include consideration of practice, genetics, and the interaction between the two.

Expertise is relative. An expert is someone who can perform better than 95 percent of people trying to do the same thing. We don't make the expertise judgment by comparing ourselves with other species. Nor do we make it across different levels of development. People are not experts at language just because dogs or babies can't talk. They are merely competent. The expertise judgment is made among people engaged in the same activity. For example, the expert base stealer does it best relative to his peers. Rickey Henderson has stolen more bases than anyone (1,406) and is clearly an expert. Bountiful baseball statistics allow us to create extremely refined versions of base-stealing expertise. We could also designate Hugh Nicol an expert because he stole the most in a single season (138), or Ty Cobb because he stole home more than anyone else (54). Endless baseball statistics make us notice how experts have set themselves apart and allow us to argue about who in this already rarified group is better.

Rather than splitting hairs this way, the bigger challenge

is to understand how expert players got as good as they did and to determine if there are common factors that led to their successes.

PRACTICE MAKES PERFECT

In an influential set of papers written between 1993 and 1996, Anders Ericsson studied the background and methods of experts with a broad range of skills. His goal was to develop a general theory of expertise that would be useful for understanding all expert performance. His approach still seems radical because it makes no distinctions between mental or physical skills and completely ignores genetic factors. This is counterintuitive for those who believe there are big differences in what it takes to be a great athlete versus a great intellect. Ericsson came to an extreme conclusion: All expertise comes from practice, and lots of it. Practice is necessary whether one desires to become the greatest chess player, accountant, radiologist, musician, or pitcher. A powerfully trained brain is needed for expert thinking or doing, and the practice requirements to get to this level of performance are the same for all brain activities. This conclusion led my colleague Rich Ivry to propose that if Michael Jordan had spent as much time studying physics as he had shooting hoops, he might have had a shot at a Nobel Prize.

Can this really be the case? Is practice the only requirement for expertise? Ericsson's main conclusion is based on the consistent observation that no expert can escape practice. Michael Jordan's daily practice throughout adolescence and high school is legendary.

A study of musicians in England established this quantitatively. It showed that the level of musicianship in people sampled randomly from the general population correlated tightly with the number of years they had practiced. The same applies for great chess players, accountants, and radiologists. Ericsson noted that having talent at an early age is far less reliable at predicting subsequent success in a sport. He found that expertise typically emerges after ten years of solid practice. Virtuoso musicians typically will have practiced about four hours a day for ten years, constituting more than twelve thousand hours total. What about baseball players? Big-league players also will have been playing the game for more than ten years by the time they make it professionally.

Does the brain change after ten years of baseball practice? There are no good data to answer this question. But it is possible to draw inferences from a rapidly emerging literature describing brain changes in musicians. One stunning fact, revealed by high-resolution pictures of the brain obtained with magnetic resonance imaging scanners, is that the motor cortex of expert musicians is larger than in novices. The motor cortex is the key part of the brain for organizing signals to activate muscles synergistically. Critically, the changes occur only in specific places. The motor cortex is organized around different parts of the body, with the leg, arm, and face areas in different locations. Only the arm area is bigger in the violinist or pianist.

One could make the argument that the musician doesn't grow this area with practice. Rather, he might play a particular instrument because he was born with a larger-than-usual area in his motor cortex. However, this argument is neutralized by recent brain anatomy studies of musicians with different years of experience. They show a relationship between motor cortex size and amount of practice.

This evidence of local brain growth with practice has profound implications for models of something called neural plasticity. We are all familiar with the idea that muscles can grow with exercise and that brains can rewire at the microscopic level to accommodate new knowledge. This new information shows the capacity of the brain to undergo large-scale reorganization at the macroscopic level. The finding raises a number of questions. Because the skull cavity for the brain is a fixed volume, enlargement of one brain area may come at the cost to another area. We do not know if the making of a great pitcher or hitter comes at the cost of doing something else. It would also be desirable to define conditions that would allow the brain to undergo similar growth after stroke or brain injury.

In parallel with structural changes, experts demonstrate differences in the way their brains activate networks of neurons to accomplish a task. Using a special type of brain scanning called functional magnetic resonance imaging, or fMRI, relative changes of local brain activity can be pinpointed. It is possible to detect brain areas that are turned on while a person executes a particular task compared to baseline, such as lying still in the scanner and relaxing. When healthy young volunteers perform a simple motor skill in the scanner, such as playing a simple arpeggio on piano keys, a distributed set of sensory and motor regions is strongly activated.

These areas are normally involved in planning a movement, making instantaneous adjustments, and sequencing finger movements in the correct order. Comparison studies between novice musicians and experts show that the experts recruit far less brain volume, even when the two groups are performing the identical movements at the same speed. Analogous results can be found in healthy people who learn a new motor skill and undergo repeated scanning over many months of practice. Early on there is a rapid increase in the volume of brain areas that are activated to perform the skill. In parallel, there is an increase in the electrical excitability of the motor cortex, which projects down to the spinal cord.

This increase is measured by stimulating the cortex with a brief magnetic pulse in what is called transcranial magnetic stimulation, or TMS. The TMS stimulator uses a coil of copper wire, bundled into a handle that looks like a thick ping-pong paddle. The handle is held against the scalp and can be adjusted over the front or back of the brain using MRI scans to guide positioning. When a brief but powerful electric current is sent through the coil of wire, a magnetic pulse is generated at the scalp and is transmitted through the skull onto the outer layers of the brain. This will excite the underlying brain for about a quarter of a second. Function in most brain areas is disrupted by this excitation. If the TMS coil is positioned over a motor area, there can be brief twitches of muscles controlled by this motor area. After a small amount of practice the same muscle twitch can be evoked with the coil positioned over a larger area of brain. This indicates a rapid change in cortical excitability as connections that would block the twitch become less active. Evoking the twitch with a less-targeted coil is a sign that the cortex is in the early stages of potential reorganization.

But after extensive practice, the reverse happens. The volume of activation steadily declines to an amount less than that in novices, and the pattern of electrical excitability induced by TMS changes shape. An additional important finding is that the volume of activation is reduced in experts only if they are performing a task that is similar to what they have practiced over the years. An expert baseball player would probably not show expertise effects in the brain while performing a piano keyboard task.

Another finding from fMRI studies is that practice leads to changes in the strength of connections between areas. This can be measured in fMRI by determining whether two areas are more likely to fire at the same time after training. Brain areas are richly interconnected, with information processing shared across many areas. Learning isn't just the turning on or turning off of local brain areas, it is a change in the neural dynamics within circuits. As areas fire together, their functional connection strengthens.

These observations support the idea that expertise is explained in part by higher cortical efficiency. The expert uses much less brain activity to do the practiced activity. The implication is that many years of practice may lead to a neural network that is highly efficient at using the fewest number of synapses to get a behavior accomplished. The rest of us might be fumbling about, calculating all sorts of solutions for a desired behavior. Inefficiency in the novice baseball player may come at a cost in terms of poor or slow planning, sensitivity to distraction, or early fatigue. This interpretation is consistent with the descriptions that experts provide on how they maximize performance.

FOCUSED INTENSITY

Mental effort and better focus on a task throughout training might very well lead to enhanced neural efficiency. Experts are widely recognized for their ability to restrict their thinking to information relevant to the task and nothing else. In baseball this is a renowned feature of great hitters: They leverage their skill of instantly recognizing and crushing a particular kind of pitch. They focus and wait for something very specific. In 2002, Barry Bonds explained to broadcaster Rick Sutcliffe that he had reduced the strike zone to a tiny hitting area, and that's all he looked at. "It's about the size of a quarter," Bonds said. In 1986, Ted Williams told Don Mattingly something similar: "Until I got to two strikes, I looked for one pitch in one area, about the size of a silver dollar." The same principle applies for pitchers. Reliever Tom Gordon was with the Cubs when he said, "I focus on making that one pitch. That's what I tell myself, one pitch. You can't worry about the next one. Even with a good hitter, he'll get out seven times out of ten. I want to make sure that this is one of those seven."

Studies of brain images are just beginning to allow researchers to examine the neural correlates of this exceptional level of mental focus. It is even possible under special circumstances to "read" people's minds with a brain scanner and predict how they will perform. In visual detection tasks, where subjects are trying to locate target objects among distractions—analogous to the "Where's Waldo" puzzle—it is possible to distinguish trials that are successful or unsuccessful simply by looking at the degree to which irrelevant brain areas are activated. The expert may learn to maintain executive control over irrelevant brain circuits that need to stay out of the way.

Another way to understand success is by considering the expert's ability to plan his actions in terms of outcomes rather than means. It is possible that novices don't have enough physical experience to plan an action in terms of an outcome. They are stuck organizing action in terms of particular movements or steps. A beginning hitter may think about elbow position, hip angle, or remembering to keep his eyes on the ball. Although the expert can also think about these specifics during training, in general, experts organize action at a higher level in terms of where the ball will go.

Recent fMRI experiments support this distinction. My colleagues and I mapped out what happens in the brain as subjects watch other people perform familiar actions, such as picking up a cup, moving a wine bottle, or opening a box. The key finding was that no single part in the brain is used to understand action. There is a cascade of interacting brain areas, with some areas mostly concerned with low-level details such as where a hand is reaching, how it is grasping, or the weight of something being lifted. At an intermediate level, different brain areas are engaged for what is being grasped or the means by which an object is manipulated. Finally, there is a higher level of brain representation related to the outcome of an action. Is the person opening a box or closing it? Is she lifting a glass to fill it or to put it away? This nested set of brain systems is also engaged in a similar cascade of function when we are planning and executing actions. Thus, at the brain level, there are distinguishable systems used for means and outcomes of motor actions. Training teaches us where in this maze of control circuitry to represent a desired action. In baseball, the implication is that the hitter visualizes a desired outcome and does not focus on swing adjustments, and the pitcher plans where the ball will go, not how the arm will move to get it there. The novice, on the other hand, has a murky idea of the relationship between the means and the outcome of an action.

What happens in brain areas that understand action in

terms of outcomes as we train someone to become an expert? Do expert baseball players "see" the actions of other players better because they can embody the other players' movements in their own nervous systems? Exciting new results from experiments with dancers support the idea that physical experience allows us to simulate another person's movements in our own heads. To test this, we had a group of modern dancers learn a new, extremely difficult dance piece over six weeks of training. Their brains were scanned once a week as they watched video clips of their teacher performing the dance piece they were learning and another piece that they didn't get to physically practice. Watching dance moves they actually practiced was more likely to engage brain areas related to understanding action in terms of outcomes. Furthermore, the better they could perform a particular movement, the more action areas were engaged when watching someone else making a similar movement. This shows that becoming an expert involves, in part, learning the meaning of an action at a more complex level of analysis for both the self and others.

SMART PRACTICE

Harry Caray, the Cubs announcer, once said, "I've only been doing this fifty-four years. With a little experience, I might get better." Even though developing expertise requires lots of practice, does extensive practice guarantee that one will become an expert? Not necessarily. There are many examples of people toiling away at a problem without major improvement. This led Ericsson and others to argue that practice needs to be smart and tailored to the individual's level of skill to maximize effective learning. Practice should also be effortful, with demands placed on the player to learn to stay on task and maintain control in difficult situations. The musician practices the hard parts of a composition. The best players learn to use their time wisely, focusing on elements most likely to enhance performance. The athlete might work on strength training, speed training, specific skills, or mental focus. Physical sports don't always require physical practice, and mental skills don't require only mental practice. In 1998, Mark McGwire raced Sammy Sosa to break the single-season home run record. McGwire spent hours each day simply watching videos of opposing pitchers: "I study pitchers. I visualize pitches. That gives me a better chance every time I step into the box. That doesn't mean I'm going to get a hit every game, but that's one of the reasons I've come a long way as a hitter."

The consequences of smart practice compared to exercise alone are beginning to be found in the brain. In rats, learning a new skill, such as traversing a rotating rod (akin to running down the length of a rolling log), leads to the growth of new neuronal connections in motor areas involved in coordination and the real-time adjustment of movement. In contrast, workouts on the running wheel in the cage lead to growth only of blood vessels that supply the brain with nutrients.

In humans, the consequences of smart practice are less well understood. Performing a basic movement such as tapping your fingers over and over will briefly change the excitability of the motor cortex. This change in excitability reflects a preparation to start to learn. But this is only the first step toward reorganization. Only with long-term practice and demands to generate new types of movements do these maps of cortical excitability change permanently.

Mixing up a practice schedule in unexpected ways can enhance effective practice. Imagine hitting against a pitching machine that is throwing curves, fastballs, or sliders. By the end of practice, you will be much better at hitting each of these types of pitches if you take them in groups (all the curves, then all the fastballs, then all the sliders) than if they are mixed up so you don't know what you will get on any given pitch. It is also a lot more fun to take the pitches in groups. Hitting unknown types of pitches takes much more concentration and effort and performance is rarely as good.

However, by the next day, a curious thing happens. The player who looked so good from the grouped practice does worse than the player who got unexpected pitches each time. This phenomenon, called contextual interference, also works for language learning, problem solving, and many sports, including golf. Functional magnetic resonance imaging studies are beginning to show the brain basis for this benefit of smart practice. My research team had subjects learn to perform different arpeggios on a keyboard, with the arpeggios presented one at a time or in a mixed distribution. Not unexpectedly, at the end of the training on the first day, performance in the mixed group was not as good. Nevertheless, more changes were taking place in motor planning areas during training in the mixed group. In another study, subjects were brought back the next day and those in the mixed group performed better, typical of the contextual interference effect. This demonstrates the brain's ability to gain additional motor memory after practice has ended. It shows that motor memories typically take time to become permanently fixed into brain circuits. After a good night of sleep, which can help "consolidate," or solidify, motor memories, the mixed group showed persistent increased activity in motor areas. These results show that judicious organization of a practice schedule can lead to increased brain plasticity and better long-term storage in motor areas.

THE COST OF TOO MUCH THINKING

During practice, a ballplayer can spend enormous amounts of time consciously evaluating his own performance, followed by making adjustments and reevaluating. There is emerging evidence that too much thinking during practice can actually interfere with learning motor skills that are better left to unconscious control. A more important goal is to learn to play automatically—that is, to play "lights out." As Yogi Berra noted, "Think!? How the hell are you gonna think and hit at the same time?"

There are a number of ways to test whether a skill has become automatic. One common approach in psychology experiments is to see whether adding a second task will hurt performance. We are all capable of driving down the open highway while talking on the cell phone, drinking a coffee, adjusting the radio, or talking to the kids in the backseat. Riding with a teenage driver reinforces the fact that safely executing this level of multitasking takes years of practice.

However, characterizing automaticity based on multitasking is a tricky approach because it is a relative definition that depends a lot on the testing environment. It is one thing to drive and talk on a cell phone on an empty highway. Driving is entirely different in city traffic where performance limits can easily be reached and a driver becomes a real hazard when performing any secondary task such as talking on the phone. This relative definition of automaticity poses a challenge for designing good brain imaging studies of automaticity based on multitasking. A central controversy in this research area is whether improvements in multitasking emerge because people get better at switching back and forth between two tasks or whether they learn to do two things simultaneously.

A big part of training in any sport is to get the player to a level of control that does not require conscious evaluation. The reason is that during a game, conscious self-evaluation is found, more often than not, to actually harm performance. A key quality of the expert is to shut down this conscious control. John Kruk, former first baseman for the Philadelphia Phillies, described his hitting strategy this way: "I try to dumb down out there. They tell you to stay within yourself, so that's what I do. Mentally, I'm not gonna out-think myself too often." One reason that self-evaluation is so bad is that it is so slow. Automatic control processes, such as the unconscious adjustment of a swing for an approaching curve ball, can occur as fast as 50 milliseconds after the shift in the ball trajectory is detected. In contrast, conscious adjustments of a swing will take four times longer. The ball will be long past the hitter in this situation.

Brain imaging studies on the neural underpinnings of motor control are identifying strong distinctions between motor memories that are learned consciously and those that are learned unconsciously. Consider experiments where people learn a simple motor skill, such as tapping out a phone number on a keyboard. Conscious memory is used to remember the phone number and the layout of a novel keypad. In parallel, unconscious memories of the finger movements needed to tap out the sequence are being burned into motor areas. Early on, the conscious memory dominates. With time and practice the unconscious memories take control and allow for fast, accurate, and automatic keying of a familiar phone number.

Many brain imaging studies now show that each of these memories is formed in a different brain area. For ballplayers, a key fact is that motor skill learning that is unconscious occurs in motor areas, whereas conscious learning is more likely to take place in areas associated with decision making or cognitive control. In recent studies, my colleagues and I have used transcranial magnetic stimulation to show that the control circuit where unconscious learning takes place is also where we adjust movements when there are unexpected changes, analogous to adjusting a baseball swing when we detect a curve ball. When subjects try to grasp an object that is changing shape and the control circuit is disrupted by TMS, the subject is unable to adjust the fingers to the new shape. Similarly, if the object changes position, they are no longer able to move the arm to the new location. Instead, the hand goes to the original shape or location using a preplanned action. Critically, this updating circuit works even when a subject is unaware that a target has moved or changed shape. Thus, we have been able to identify the key circuits that ballplayers use for rapid, online control of motor performance, which operate at an unconscious level.

We could easily redefine expertise as effortless grace. As Cubs second baseman Manny Trillo once noted, "There's no trying in baseball. You either go out and do it, or you don't." Whereas an average player might benefit from willfully trying harder, or "giving it 110 percent," the expert always seems beyond all that. In addition, trying to win or to break a record can create a distraction and interfere with the task at hand. Cubs manager Don Baylor said of being hit by 267 pitches— then a record—"I was up there to get a hit. I wasn't trying to get hit." One way neuroscientists think about this phenomenon is with resource models of brain processing. Trying to break a record costs our brain time and energy that would be better spent focusing on the pitcher.

Every player or team is at risk of losing in a clutch situation. One possible explanation is that performance declines are just part of the normal variation that any athlete will experience. Another possibility is that a player or team is actually "choking," or collapsing under pressure. Coaches don't like the idea that an expert athlete could actually choke. After a particularly rough season, Dusty Baker, the manager of the Cubs, exclaimed, "Did Florida choke? Did Philly choke? Does that make everybody who didn't win a choker? . . . I've never had a team that's described as 'choked.' So I'm not going to have one now." Despite Baker's denial, there is good statistical evidence to show that expert teams can choke and that they are more likely to choke in a home game, in front of a friendly crowd, during the semifinals or league championship.

The cost of trying too hard while executing motor skills might explain what happens when a player or entire team chokes. In a home game the player is trying to make the fans or teammates happy, resulting in a shift in focus to the outcome of the game at a cost in performance. In these situations errors start to compound as the players lose focus. Cubs fans already are thinking of their team's meltdown during the 2003 National League Championship Series. Arguably, the deciding play was not when a fan caught a foul ball that might have been playable but the shortstop's error that followed. In an away game, the crowd may be hostile and loud, but players are free of the need to please, which may help them focus on hitting or fielding.

In contrast to choking, where an expert player or team

focuses too much on external pressures such as the crowd, panic has been characterized as an inability to distribute attention to all aspects of the game. Panic happens when inexperienced players focus too much on one detail in a game. A hitter might be attending to a teammate's lead off first base, or a relief pitcher might be overly concerned with the number of opponents on base. Experts keep from getting caught up in distractions. Cubs relief pitcher Matt Karchner underscored his ability to keep from panicking with the bases loaded this way: "I don't care. Just give me the ball. Relievers are trained to react. We're like dogs."

INNER DRIVE

Given the central role of effortful, long-term practice in creating brilliance in sports, it is all too clear that motivation may ultimately be the critical ingredient for success. Unfortunately, motivation is still a magic potion that few coaches, parents, or teachers understand. Famous Cub Ernie Banks understood at least part of the recipe when he was a coach: "I like my players to be married and in debt. That's the way you motivate them."

Neuroscientists haven't added much to this model. We know a lot about motivation in relationship to immediate rewards such as money and sex and what it takes to get a person to work harder for these short-term gains. Consider the brain activity of a gambler in Las Vegas. We can readily create gambling conditions during brain imaging experiments and examine the situations under which a person will most likely want to repeat an action, such as making another bet in a slot machine, upping an ante, or taking foolish risks. A key finding in rats, monkeys, and humans is that games where the rewards are entirely unpredictable are the best at inducing a person to make another bet. This unpredictability leads to maximal release of dopamine, a key brain chemical involved in decision making and normal learning. Without it we can't make up our minds, take chances, or discover through exploration. The flip side is that it is also involved in dysfunctional behaviors such as pathological gambling and drug addiction. At this point we can only speculate that dopamine and related neurochemical systems used for immediate gains also form the basis of the type of motivation or drive that leads a kid to practice long and hard over many years. The ultimate ingredient needed for success was captured best by Sammy Sosa during his 1998 quest for the single-season home run record: "I'm not going to lie to you—I'm having a good time."

GENES AND NATURAL TALENT

An alternate model of expertise is that it is dependent on the endowment of good genes. As long as there have been measures of neural signals there have been attempts to link genes, nervous system physiology, and performance. In 1929, a Professor Kato at Keio University in Tokyo (then spelled "Tokio") figured out how to measure the information-carrying speed of nerves in the arms or legs of people. He immediately applied it to athletes. His work was featured in a July 2, 1929, *New York Times* article (see sidebar). Kato found that Ty Cobb's nerves relayed signals at three miles a minute, possibly faster than normal. At that time, nerve speed was considered immutable. Thus, the implication was that Cobb was born with fast nerves that gave him a unique advantage for hitting and running. This example captures an intuition widely held in our culture that being a great athlete is invariably associated with being born with good genes.

Says Nerve Reponses Go 3 Miles a Minute

Professor Kato Holds Superior Brain Is Secret
to Ty Cobb's and Bobby Jones's Success.

Special to the New York Times   *July 2, 1929*

Baltimore, Md., July 1—Messages from eye to brain and from brain to hand travel three miles a minute, says Professor G. Kato of Keio University, Tokio, Japan, authority on nerve construction research, who is visiting the Johns Hopkins Medical School here. According to Dr. Kato, it is not Ty Cobb's batting eye or Bobby Jones's master touch or Thurston's slight of hand, but the brain that makes the difference.

For years in his laboratory at the Physiological Institute at Keio, of which he is director, Professor Kato has been conducting the delicate experiments on the nerve fibre of the Japanese toad. He said:

"In the course of these experiments we made the astonishing discovery that as the temperature of the toad increased to that of the room in which the experiments were being made the speed of the nerve reaction increased."

"We cut down the temperature and the speed diminished. We raised the toad's nerve fibre to the temperature of the human body and found that the speed of the nerve impulse was exactly the same as that of human fibre, sixty-three meters a second—three miles a minute."

The brain, he said, is divided into two areas, the sensory and the motor. The motor portion delivers commands through the nerve fibers by a chemical and electrical process to the muscles, which obey, he explained, and the sensory portion receives, by the same chemical and electrical process, the various senses of sight, hearing and feeling.

"Everybody," he commented, "does not have a brain that can transfer those impulses from one-half of the brain to the other in just exactly the same way that Cobb's brain does. That is what makes the difference between one person's performance and another's.

"In golf the same is true. The control of the player over his club is the result of nerve impulses traveling constantly between brain and hand and hand and brain. The performance, whether good or bad, depends upon what goes on within the brain cells; not, as so many think, upon the nerves and muscles."

There has been a recurring hope that simple genetic inheritance, based on the expression of single genes, might explain biological properties that make us experts. Clearly, single mutations of genes can lead to abnormal development, cancer, or metabolic disease. However, the flip side is rarely if ever true. It is unlikely that we will find examples where single gene mutations lead to increased capacity to develop expertise. We are currently in the midst of a second wave of discovery in molecular genetics in which all DNA in a single person can be mapped and sufficient information is available to compare genes across populations of people. This science supports the proposition that genes do matter in developing expertise, but the patterning of genetic information needed to create great athletes is extremely complicated, with involvement of many genes and gene-environment interactions.

Characterizing the genetic factors that make someone more likely to succeed in baseball will probably take decades. The first big problem is that baseball demands many skills and there are lots of ways to find success in the game, from being a power hitter to a fastball pitcher to a (weak-hitting) defensive specialist, each linked to particular body morphologies and brain function. Second, genetics is complicated. Genetic expression is modulated by development, experience, and learning in a dynamic interplay between environment and organism.

This modulation of genetic expression is essential for learning in the brain. This critical area in genetics may ultimately play a central role for understanding the formation of expertise, based on the study of genes and what are called transcription factors during development and practice. Transcription factors are proteins that respond to biological signals and change the rate at which genes are turned on and off in cells. Thus, they regulate when and how much particular proteins are made. The genes themselves are not changed by these factors. As the ballplayer develops, practice and experience might lead to different genetic expression, with changes in brain and body tightly coupled to what was practiced. The recognition that the body is constantly remaking itself at the cellular level provides an escape route from the false dichotomy that expertise emerges exclusively from either practice or genetics. Experience changes genetic expression, which changes the person.

Even in cases where genetics do appear to be essential for sports success, it is rare to find examples were genes are the only thing that matters. One of the best examples of a physiologic measure that is determined almost entirely by a complex set of genetic factors and that is critical for determining success in endurance sports is the VO_2 max. This is a measure of how efficiently a person can move oxygen through the lungs and into the bloodstream, where it can be used to make energy for nerves and muscles. Elite bicyclists such as Lance Armstrong are born with genes giving them a value that is 30 to 50 percent greater than what the rest of us have. Exercise and training can change our VO_2 a little bit, but never enough to catch up with Lance. Similar findings hold true for the proportion of fast- versus slow-twitch muscle fibers. Our genes give us a proportion that can be modified only modestly by training. Professional athletes can have a higher percentage of one type or the other. Sprinters may have as much as 80 percent fast-twitch fibers and long-distance runners may have as much as 80 percent slow-twitch fibers. These differences of VO_2 and muscle type strongly constrain the types of sports where a person, endowed with a relatively inflexible physiology, could find success. But even in these well-defined examples, it is clear that good genes and physiology alone don't assure success. For example, differences between the VO_2 max for the top riders in the Tour de France are negligible. At that level of performance, other physical and mental factors based on strategic training, strong motivation, and effective strategy define success.

Back at the ballpark, your daughter and her team are down by three and starting to deflate a little. You start to wonder if her generation, when she becomes a parent, will have sufficient information about genetic expression and regulation to be able to develop predictive tests for skills as complicated as baseball. Given the complexity of the game, this still seems pretty far-fetched. In the meantime, she is just going to have to follow the advice of Bill Buckner, offered when he was the Chicago Cubs' first baseman: "There's nothing wrong with this team that more hitting, more pitching, more fielding, and more hitting couldn't help."

-3-

WHY DID CASEY STRIKE OUT?

The Neuroscience of Hitting

JOHN MILTON, M.D., PH. D., F.R.C.P.C.,

ANA SOLODKIN, PH.D.,

AND STEVEN L. SMALL, PH.D., M.D.

> *The sneer is gone from Casey's lip, his teeth are clinched in hate;*
> *He pounds with cruel violence his bat upon the plate.*
> *And now the pitcher holds the ball, and now he lets it go,*
> *And now the air is shattered by the force of Casey's blow.*

E. L. Thayer, "Casey at the Bat" (1888)

The focal point of baseball is the confrontation between batter and pitcher. Consequently, a great deal of effort has been devoted to discovering the hidden truths of baseball through analyses of the biomechanics of throwing and hitting, the physical laws that govern the movements of the ball and bat, and the statistics of baseball's successes and failures.

However, the play of baseball is not solely determined

by physics, chance, and the three S's of athletic ability: size, strength, and speed. It is also heavily influenced by the effects of novel game situations on the ability of the player's nervous system to make good decisions, plans, and executions. Here we view the batter–pitcher duel from the point of view of the neural networks involved in making the motor programs that enable the batter to swing the bat. We show that there is more to hitting a baseball than meets the eye.

RESPONSE TIMES

An absolute truth in baseball is that for a hit to occur, the bat and the ball must arrive at the same spot at the same time. This fact motivates analyses of hitting in terms of response times; i.e., does the batter have enough time to respond once the ball is pitched? In order to answer this question we need to compare the time it takes the ball to travel from the pitcher's hand to home plate with the time it takes the batter's nervous system to detect the direction and speed of the ball, plan the response, and then execute the body movements that enable hitting the ball. Although this may seem to be a difficult task, we can actually obtain some useful insights by making some simple calculations.

Where to begin? Well, the distance from the pitching mound to home plate is sixty feet, six inches. However, we need to account for the decrease in this distance accounted for by the forward step and outstretched arm of the pitcher as the ball is delivered. Let's assume that the forward step and outstretched arm of the pitcher's delivery reduce the distance that the ball travels by six feet. This means that we need to determine how much time it takes for the baseball to travel fifty-four feet, six inches.

Physics tells us that time is equal to distance divided by speed. Pitchers vary the speed of their pitches in order to "keep batters on their toes," and thus we need to estimate the range of times that embraces all of the different pitches that a pitcher can throw. In the major leagues the speed of a pitched ball likely varies between about 60 and 100 miles per hour. By performing the math we see that it takes 0.367 seconds (fastest pitch) to 0.614 seconds (slowest pitch) for the baseball to travel between the pitcher's hand and home plate. For most of us armchair athletes this is less than the time between successive heartbeats.

Now we need to figure out how much time it takes the batter to react and swing the bat. Estimates suggest that the time it takes elite baseball hitters to respond to the pitched ball—their response time—is in the neighborhood of 0.33 seconds. Because this is less time than it takes the ball to travel to home plate (0.367–0.614 seconds), it is tempting to think that the secret of success is simply a matter of learning to have a fast response time. However, how does the batter figure out what speed the pitch is traveling? A swing that is too fast relative to the ball speed means that the hitter will be "out in front of the pitch" and hence either pull the ball foul or miss the pitch altogether, especially if the pitcher is throwing a sinker.

A trick scientists use when they don't know what is going on is to make an educated guess, or hypothesis, that they can then test. Baseball fans might be surprised to learn that scientists often hope their hypotheses eventually turn out to be wrong, because the necessity of making a new hypothesis provides an opportunity to learn something new. For example, let's hypothesize that the batter's brain decides whether to swing at the ball or not, then makes the program to tell the muscles what to do so that the body swings the bat. This is called a sequential model because the steps—making a decision, planning what to do, and then executing that plan—occur independently, one after the other, with no overlap.

We can evaluate whether this sequential model provides a good description of the interplay between batter and pitcher by examining how it would be possible for a batter to learn to lower his response time. The hitter's response time includes a brain part and a muscle part. According to our educated guess, we can add these two components in order to come up with overall response time. Thus, one way for the hitter to lower the total response time is to do exercises that will decrease the time it takes to complete his swing. Estimates of muscle response time for a baseball swing are of the order of 0.18 to 0.25 seconds. However, it is unlikely that a batter could improve his muscle response by more than a few milliseconds, even with a great deal of practice. As we will soon see, such small reductions in muscle response are unlikely to produce a significant change in hitting prowess.

The second possibility is that hitting ability is related to factors involved in determining the time it takes the hitter's brain to figure out what to do. If we take a conservative estimate of 0.25 seconds for the muscle response in a hitter's swing, then we can subtract that from the overall response time to figure out the brain's response time. We arrive at an answer of 0.08 seconds.

It takes about 0.043 seconds for information concerning the velocity and trajectory of the baseball to be sent from the retina of the eye to higher areas of the visual cortex in the brain. This means that the hitter's brain would have only 0.037 seconds available to interpret the type of pitch (fastball, curveball) and plan all of the motor activities necessary to swing the bat.

That sounds too good to be true, and indeed it is. Even under optimal conditions of attention, adults age twenty-eight or twenty-nine—the years of peak hitting performance—can respond to a sensory stimulus, such as a randomly flashing light, in no less than 0.2 seconds, more than five times longer than our estimate for baseball hitters. Moreover, because response time increases as the complexity of the task increases, we can anticipate that, in game situations, hitters' response times will likely be much longer.

These observations demonstrate that our sequential model for the interplay between pitcher and hitter is not possible. This same conclusion has been reached by scientists who study other fast-ball sports as well, including cricket, soccer, tennis, field hockey, and volleyball. This realization has greatly limited the usefulness of estimates of response times for analyzing a baseball hitter's performance. A second problem with equating hitting skill with response time is the implication that hitters with slow response times would never be able to hit a fastball, a theory that runs contrary to observation. Our brief scientific investigation leads us to the unmistakable conclusion that neural planning for hitting must, at least in part, occur concurrently with the swing itself.

In fact, deciding and planning begin even before the ball leaves the pitcher's hand. Let's see how it is possible for the baseball hitter's brain to buy this extra time.

READING THE WINDUP

What is the nature of the information that the batter uses to make decisions about swinging his bat? Recent research emphasizes that athletes in fast-ball sports anticipate where the ball will be based on kinematically relevant sources of information. In baseball, this information is gathered before the ball is thrown: a batter may note the movements the pitcher makes during the windup, remember his past experiences with this pitcher, and pick up clues from watching the pitcher face previous batters.

Two observations in cricket batters underscore the importance of anticipatory clues for hitting performance. First, suppose we showed a batter only the windup that a pitcher makes without showing him the flight of the ball and where it ended up in the catcher's mitt. How well can the hitter predict where the ball will go? One study found that expert cricket batters were much better judges about the type, speed, and location of the pitch about to be thrown than weak batters. Second, skilled batters perform better against human cricket pitchers (who are called *bowlers*) than a mechanical bowling machine that provides no advance information concerning movement pattern.

A clear relationship exists between the skill level of the batter and the type of information that is extracted in this pre-swing period. It is not simply the case that a good batter extracts the same information as a poor batter but in a better way. The good batter actually extracts highly relevant information for the task that the poor batter does not. For example, expert cricket batsmen focus on specific bowling hand and arm cues that novices tend to overlook. This same trend—i.e., that the type of information extracted by experts is more focused than that extracted by novices—is also seen in other fast-ball sports, such as by goalkeepers during the soccer penalty shot.

THE SPACE BETWEEN THE BATTER'S EARS

The striking feature of fast-ball sports, such as baseball, is that the length of time available for the batter's brain to formulate a good anticipation of the pitch and its location is much longer (at least seconds) than the time that it takes for the batter to make the swing (milliseconds). This pre-swing period has its counterpart in the aiming sports, such as archery, rifle shooting, and golf, where it is called the pre-shot routine. Thus, what appear to distinguish a good athlete from a poor athlete in these sports are the activities that occur within the six-inch space between the batter's ears, in the batter's brain. What are the neural systems that are active during this preparatory period, and do they differ as a function of skill level?

In order to successfully hit the pitched ball, the hitter's brain must be involved in two tasks: (1) preparing the neural programs for the movements involved in swinging the bat and (2) interpreting the movements of the pitcher in order to predict where the pitched ball will go. Although it is quite likely that these two tasks occur simultaneously, we will describe what is known about them separately.

PREPARING TO SWING

Modern methods of brain imaging, particularly functional magnetic resonance imaging (fMRI), have made it possible to peer inside an athlete's brain while he is preparing to swing a bat. Using fMRI it is possible to detect specific brain regions that are more active while a subject performs one type of task compared to another. Because the subject is inside an MRI machine, he cannot actually swing a bat. However, fMRI does allow us to detect those areas that are most active while athletes are in the motor preparation phase—the pre-swing routine—provided that they can properly imagine preparing for and performing the swing without actually swinging. Although fMRI has not yet been used to study hitting a baseball, such studies have been conducted for novice and expert golfers preparing to hit a golf ball. We anticipate that observations will be similar in baseball hitters during their pre-swing routine.

Figure 1 compares the fMRI of a novice golfer and an expert golfer as they visualize a golf scene and prepare to swing the golf club compared to when they visualize similar non-golf scenes and do not prepare to swing. There are a number of surprising observations. First of all, the novice player tends to have more brain activation than the expert. This may sound counterintuitive because it is easy to suppose that more is better. However, not only this study but others as well have shown this same phenomenon over and over: well-trained subjects (not only human) have less brain activation than beginners when performing comparable tasks. This has been interpreted to mean that, in professionals, the efficiency of the brain for a particular skill increases with training. In the end, less brain work is required to perform the task (and as we know, the task is performed much better).

Second, as was observed in cricket batters, not only is the brain of the novice golfer working harder when doing the same tasks as the expert, but the novice appears to be trying to solve a more complex task. In our study, expert golfers activated only those brain regions critically necessary for performing the task: regions involved in motor planning (labeled CMA, SMA, PM in figure 1), seeing the ball (OCC in figure 1),

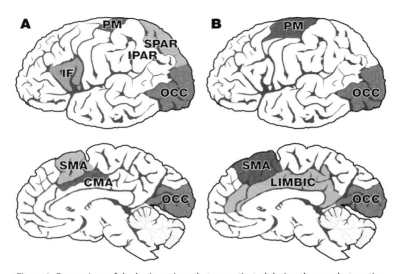

Figure 1. Comparison of the brain regions that are activated during the pre-shot routine of an expert golfer (A) and a novice golfer (B). *Abbreviations:* CMA: cingulate motor, IF: inferior frontal, IPAR: inferior parietal, LIMBIC: limbic (note that the amygdala region cannot be seen in this view), PM: premotor, OCC: occipital cortex, SMA: supplementary motor, SPAR: superior parietal. The primary motor cortex is located within a region called the sulcus, just posterior to the PM region. The mirror neurons are located within the IF region. Courtesy of Ana Solodkin and John Milton. Adapted by William Stilwell.

and those involved in and relating visual input to motor planning (SPAR in figure 1).

However, novices activate additional brain regions that are not activated in experts. In particular, novices activate several of the so-called limbic regions, which are thought to constitute the neural foundation of emotion. This activation of limbic regions, such as the amygdala and basal forebrain complex, is quite intriguing because of the association with emotional control and autonomic control (i.e., the brain control of highly automated physiological systems, such as those involved in regulating the heart rate). A possible interpretation of the activation seen in limbic regions of novices is that the emotional content during the pre-shot routine is higher in this group than in experts. Certainly, fear and anxiety contribute to the deterioration in performance observed when athletes are placed in stressful situations, and this may be the case to some extent in these novices. In fact, both fear and anxiety have been associated with the amygdala. However, it is not clear to what extent a pre-shot routine in an MRI scanner evokes the same emotions as in the natural environment. A more likely explanation is that these responses are related to the roles played by the amygdala–basal forebrain complex in motor imagery of the imagined movement. Thus, the higher activation seen in novices relates to their increased efforts to imagine the required movement.

Interestingly, novices also activate limbic regions that are not associated with control and regulation of emotions per se, such as the posterior cingulate gyrus and nearby areas. The posterior cingulate region has been associated with functions that are important for integrating visuomotor activity with memories of previous and related movements in terms of the spatial locations of body parts (topographic memory) and their associated movements (topokinetic memory). Most important, because of its strategic location the posterior cingulate is ideally placed to focus the amount of attention that the brain should place on different sensory inputs as it plans the motor response. Indeed, it has been suggested that activation of the limbic regions, in particular the posterior cingulate, arises because the novice experiences difficulty filtering out irrelevant information. This interpretation suggests that novices hit poorly because by attending to irrelevant information they actually make the neural programming much more complex and hence less efficient than that of the experts. As we will see, this interpretation also provides the pitcher with strategies to counteract the advantages that a good hitter appears to have.

Understanding the Movements of Others

Our conclusion that neural planning for the baseball swing occurs concurrently with the swing is difficult to reconcile with the observations in figure 1 that the areas of the brain that plan motor movements (PM, IF, SMA, CMA) are not located in the same regions of the brain where visual information has traditionally been located (SPAR, OCC). In the 1980s a possible solution to this paradox was obtained through an intriguing and serendipitous discovery by Giacomo Rizzolatti. He described what was subsequently named the mirror system. Using electrophysiological recordings from the cerebral cortex of awake monkeys, Rizzolatti's group showed that one particular area of the brain contained neurons that fired when the monkey made specific goal-directed movements of the mouth or hand. This visually responsive brain region is located within IF (see figure 1); i.e., one of the brain regions involved in motor planning.

This was not too surprising. The surprise came when it was discovered that some of these neurons were active when *another* monkey performed the same goal-oriented movements with the mouth or hand. Hence the term "mirror" was coined to describe the fact that the same neurons would be similarly active whether a monkey performed a goal-oriented movement itself *or* it saw another monkey (or even a human) performing the same movement. Since Rizzolatti's discovery, the preferred hypothesis has been that mirror neurons, working together with neurons located in the inferior parietal cortex (IPAR in figure 1), play important roles both in action recognition and action understanding (hence the name *mirror system*).

Interestingly, although the functions of these neurons were first demonstrated in monkeys, recent brain imaging studies suggest that humans have a similar mirror system. Thus, it is possible to infer the roles that the different neurons in IF play as the mind of the batter prepares to hit the pitch.

Mirror neurons discharge when the batter either throws the ball or observes the pitcher throwing the ball. Hence, these neurons reflect the observed action by the motor representation encoded by the neuron of the observer. By mirroring the pitcher's movement, these neurons enable the batter to understand the subtle preparation movements of the pitcher and better anticipate the final movement and where the ball will go. How can we know this? If mirror neurons are responsible for action recognition, then these neurons should discharge when the goal of an action can be inferred, even when the action sequence itself cannot be seen. This is indeed the case. Thus, the mirror system provides the mechanism that allows the batter to predict where the ball will be having seen only a portion of the pitcher's motion.

Thus, in principle, by understanding the subtle movements involved in the motor preparations of the pitcher, using the mirror system the hitter can predict the type of ball that he will be receiving before the ball leaves the pitcher's hand. Presumably, this ability may give him additional time to prepare his own swing. This may explain the fact that a great pitcher, Babe Ruth, was also one of the greatest home run hitters of all time.

THE DUEL

Up until now we have taken a one-sided view of the confrontation between pitcher and batter. Everything seems to be in the batter's favor. Indeed, the pitcher faces a real problem since his windup actually provides essential information to the batter, which helps him anticipate where the pitched ball will go—exactly what the pitcher doesn't want to happen. Unfortunately, it is not possible for the pitcher to throw a fastball without a windup. Estimates of the power required to throw a fastball are of the order of 3–4 horsepower. It takes about a pound of muscle to generate one-eighth of a horsepower; i.e., 24–32 pounds of muscle to generate 3–4 horsepower. The muscles that are big enough to generate this amount of horsepower are located not in the arm but in the lower back and thighs of the pitcher. Thus, the windup is a necessary part of the process. In science we would call it a kinematic sequence, one that transfers power from where it is generated to the point at which it is applied—in this case, to the ball.

What is the pitcher to do? Some pitchers are able to throw pitches whose location cannot be readily related to the windup, such as a knuckleball. However, the pitcher's main weapons are deception and distraction. The neural programs inside the hitter's brain will work best if the hitter attends only to the most relevant information (see "The Cost of Too Much Thinking" in Chapter 2). Thus, the pitcher strives to mask the relevant information.

One way to do this is to provide irrelevant information. For example, since the batter is trying to pick up clues from the pitcher's windup, the pitcher can make small changes to the windup to disguise the type of pitch that he is throwing. Even slight changes to the rhythm of the windup, or an occasional step away from the mound, may be enough to cause the batter to make a small error in judgment. A pitcher who can throw with either arm, such as Greg Harris of the Montreal Expos, has the advantage that most hitters will not know enough about his two different windups to be able to make good anticipations. This fact supports professional baseball's rule against changing throwing arms while facing a batter.

Distractions are particularly useful. Extra maneuvers can provide so much irrelevant information that the working memory of the batter is overwhelmed or the batter attends to the wrong task. For example, after nearly getting hit by a fastball the batter may be more concerned about being hit than about hitting the next pitch. A batter might also be distracted by suspicion that the pitcher is doctoring the ball. Thus, a pitcher who occasionally doctors the ball can gain great mileage out of merely pretending to do so. A batter may focus attention on looking for clues to support this hypothesis, thus reducing his focus on hitting the ball. Gaylord Perry was the premier artist of this particular strategy.

By extending this line of reasoning we see that there is actually an inner game of baseball that involves not only batter and pitcher but the players and coaches of both teams. The battlefield is not only between the foul lines but also in the neural substrates that govern the activities of the players. Just as the offense maneuvers to keep the neural resources of the batter focused on hitting, the defense tries to overwhelm these resources by pulling his attention elsewhere and by providing irrelevant information. Thus, we can begin to see that there is much more to the shifting of player positions, false starts of the base runners, pauses, and the constant banter of the infielders during a baseball game than was first apparent.

CASEY STRIKES OUT!

Why did Casey strike out? From a brain perspective we can suggest several possibilities: he ignored the first two pitches (no contribution to anticipatory skill), he was angry (irrelevant information), and he played to the crowd (distraction of attention). The take-home message from Casey's fate is not that he struck out but that hitting requires not just muscle strength but also a focused, fine-tuned brain.

- 4 -

CURSES!

TOM VALEO AND LINDSAY BEYERSTEIN*

Legend has it that a billy goat—more specifically, the ejection of a man who had brought his pet goat to Wrigley Field for a World Series game in 1945—is responsible for the Chicago Cubs' inability even to reach the World Series since. Most Cubs fans are well aware of the "Curse of the Billy Goat," which is just one among many supposed curses befalling professional sports teams around the world.

In addition, athletes in every sport wear lucky socks, avoid unlucky numbers, and engage in other forms of magical thinking intended to give them a competitive edge. (See the sidebar on page 62 for examples of these and more baseball superstitions.)

There's just one catch: No scientific evidence exists for

---

*With Dan Gordon. Special thanks to Bruce Hood.

In memory of Barry Beyerstein, whose scholarship and skepticism remain a constant source of inspiration. —LB these sports-ready superstitions—or others we are wont to believe. In the 1980s, a U.S. National Research Council panel commissioned to investigate all manner of psychic events concluded that 130 years of scientific research had revealed no scientific basis for phenomena such as extrasensory perception or exercises supposed to demonstrate "mind over matter."

What, then, makes our brains liable to accept that these superstitions are real? Science does offer some answers to this question.

Cognitive neuroscientist Michael Gazzaniga's studies in split-brain patients—people who have had the corpus callosum, which connects the brain's hemispheres, severed as a treatment for epilepsy—have provided hard evidence for the idea that the brain must come up with an explanation for everything, and it will make up stories to cope with phenomena it cannot otherwise account for.

Gazzaniga has written about a split-brain subject to whom he showed different pictures—one to each side of the brain. The right side saw a snow-covered house, the left saw a chicken claw. Neither side knew what the other side saw. His patient, when asked to choose an object that matched the scenes, picked a rooster with his right hand to go with the chicken claw and a snow shovel with his left hand to go with the snowy house.

That left him with two different objects. But the left side of his brain—the side responsible for interpreting our world—was quick to reconcile his hands' different choices by concocting the explanation that he chose the shovel because it could be used to clean the chicken coop.

Moreover, Gazzaniga writes that a particular part of the brain's left hemisphere, which he calls the interpreter, is responsible for composing a continuing narrative about our beliefs and how we perceive ourselves.

Anthropologists and psychologists have written specifically about superstition in baseball, and their notions are compatible with the more general ideas neuroscience offers. George Gmelch, an anthropologist who wrote a paper called "Superstition and Ritual in American Baseball," has a unique perspective: he played baseball in the Detroit Tigers' farm system. Baseball players are particularly susceptible to superstition because they have so little control over their fate, Gmelch says. They embrace magical thinking because players are much like members of a primitive tribe—they are trying to create a sense of control over a situation fraught with uncertainty. Trobriand Islanders, for example, never performed rituals before fishing in a serene, landlocked lagoon, but before facing the dangers of the open sea they engaged in elaborate rituals intended to ensure their safe return with an abundant catch.

Most high-performance athletes have some kind of pregame routine. Coaches and sports psychologists often encourage players to develop a consistent pattern of physical and mental warm-up before a game, and many players claim that the routine helps them prepare without becoming nervous or tense. Some people play soothing music to calm themselves; others blast heavy metal to get themselves fired up.

Some psychologists maintain that even outright superstitions may still produce benefit through one of the brain's most mysterious quirks: the placebo effect. If you believe those socks will improve your performance, chances are you'll play with more confidence, which may result in a better performance.

Players' superstitions

Wade Boggs won five batting titles during his seventeen-year career and retired in 1999 with a lifetime batting average of .328, one of the highest in modern major league history. How did he do it? Some might credit his talent and his dedication to the game.

Boggs himself, however, would more likely credit the chicken he ate before each game; or his habit of leaving for the ballpark at exactly 1:47 for a 7:05 game; or fielding exactly 150 ground balls during infield practice; or his post-practice ritual of stepping on third base, second base, and first base (in that order), and then stepping on the baseline, followed by two quick steps in the coaching box before jogging off the field. He also drew the Hebrew word for life into the dirt of the batter's box before each turn at bat. He believed that helped too.

Superstition thrives in the major leagues. Boggs stood out only because his displays of magical thinking were so numerous and conspicuous, but other examples abound.

• Texas Rangers pitcher Mike Griffin's pre-game ritual eventually grew until it began a full day before with him washing his hair. Then he would eat bacon for lunch on the day of the game. While dressing for the game he would inspect his two stirrup socks and put the longer one on his right leg. While on the mound he would take off his cap after each pitch, and, like most major leaguers, he would insist on sitting on the same spot on the dugout bench.

• Infielder Julio Gotay used to play with a cheese sandwich in his back pocket.

• Pitcher Turk Wendell always wore a necklace made out of teeth from animals he had killed.

• Cleveland Indians first baseman Mike Hargrove performed so many little batting rituals that his teammates called him "the human rain delay."

• Pitcher Frank Viola used to kick up dirt exactly four times on the pitcher's mound before each pitch. If that stopped working, he'd switch to three times, or five. And in 1984, when pitching for the Minnesota Twins, he noticed that he seemed to pitch better when a fan in the bleachers unfurled a banner that read, "Frankie Sweet Music Viola." When the Twins made the World Series in 1987, Viola obtained tickets so that fan could attend both games he pitched. Yes, Viola won both.

Watch any game on TV and you'll see players display all manner of twitches, quirks, and eccentric behaviors. Pitchers tug at the bills of their caps, brush their fingers across their chests, and fidget incessantly between pitches. Batters pull on their batting gloves, kick the dirt when they step into the batter's box, and tap their helmets. Some of these gestures merely dissipate nervous energy, but some are intended to bring good luck.

Players also observe taboos, designed to avoid bad luck. Many avoid stepping on the foul line, for example. And even Little Leaguers know they should *never* mention that the pitcher has a no-hitter going. Yankee pitcher Don Larsen encountered this taboo during his perfect game against the Brooklyn Dodgers in the 1956 World Series. Midway through the game his teammates started to shun him. Although his completion of the perfect game might have reaffirmed his teammates' notions, Larsen himself wasn't buying it.

"I didn't believe in superstition," Larsen told an Associated Press reporter years later. "I was more uncomfortable the last few innings because no one would talk to me or sit next to me. The only time I was happy was when I was on the mound."

INTUITIVE REASONING

Bruce Hood, a developmental psychologist whose interests include cognitive neuroscience and magical reasoning, argues that superstition is an offshoot of normal brain function for the following reasons:

- The brain is designed to process and fill in missing information from a complex world of input.
- Understanding and predicting the world requires generating intuitive theories that infer invisible mechanisms to explain our experiences.
- Normal intuitive theories can bias rational individuals toward irrational reasoning.
- Not only are supernatural beliefs unavoidable (since they are anchored to normal intuitive theories), but these beliefs may confer beneficial effects by giving us a sense of control and purpose, perhaps even enhancing our creativity.

As humans, we are constantly looking for causes to explain the effects we see in the world, and superstitious beliefs may result from misperceiving these cause-and-effect relationships. A player who hits well may decide that his new socks had something to do with his performance and wear them in every game. Gmelch notes that a ballplayer, knowing that his skill level on a 4-for-4 day is not appreciably different than it was when he went 0-for-4 the night before, might decide that certain actions brought him good luck.

In this respect people are much like pigeons, according to psychologist B. F. Skinner. The hard-line behaviorist once conducted an experiment that he believed demonstrated superstition in the pigeon, as he put it in the title of his paper. Pigeons were placed in a cage attached to a machine that deposited food at regular intervals. The birds started to associate the food with whatever action they happened to be performing when the food last appeared. Then they would repeat that action. One made a habit of turning counter-clockwise; another learned to thrust its head into the upper corners of the cage.

Thus the pigeons appeared to be engaging in a form of superstition analogous to the rituals humans practice in hopes of gaining influence over unpredictable outcomes. Players who have a base hit in mind when they undertake elaborate batter's-box rituals will be glad to know that their actions are not unlike those of a rotating pigeon.

Indeed, more recent experiments have revealed that humans are prone to behave much like Skinner's pigeons. Japanese psychologist Koichi Ono has demonstrated this with experiments that invite people to earn reward points by pushing a lever or pressing keys on a keyboard. Even though the points were assigned randomly and had no correlation to the levers pulled or the keys tapped, many subjects repeated the behaviors that preceded a reward, as though that behavior had something to do with earning points. These superstitious beliefs often took the form of elaborate behaviors such as jumping or touching walls—behaviors they began after a coincidental increase in their scores.

In 1987, two researchers at the University of Kansas attempted a similar experiment with three- to six-year-olds. Each was left alone in a room and monitored through a one-way mirror. The room contained a clown doll called "Bobo," which dispensed marbles from his mouth either every 15 or every 30 seconds. Each child was given a box to collect marbles. A certain number of marbles would earn the child a toy.

Seventy-five percent of the children developed distinctively superstitious actions such as swinging their hips, kissing Bobo, grimacing at him, and touching his nose. Each of the children tended to repeat these behaviors over multiple sessions.

THE WAY THINGS WORK

Psychologists have proposed that superstitious beliefs are an offshoot of our conceptions—often accurate—about how things work. Any example of supernatural belief can be viewed as a misinterpretation of the available evidence or as the assumption of patterns, forces, or essences when in fact none exist. In other words, those who infer supernatural activity are detecting order and structure in the incoming information when there may be, in fact, only simple noise.

Moreover, the brain cannot handle random patterns. We see shapes in the clouds and notice rocks that look like faces or outlines of states. Likewise, because of our stubborn tendency to see outcomes as being connected to the events that precede them, we have a hard time accepting that sequential events are not causally related. Our brains are designed to learn from experience, with memories divided into fragments so we can retrieve the appropriate piece and apply it to a situation at hand. Such memory retrieval might be quite sensible: A batter with a two-strike count against a particular pitcher may recall that in the same situation three weeks ago, the pitcher threw a curveball and struck him out. However, it also makes it easy for the brain to cook up ridiculous reasoning: The last time this team made the World Series, a man and his billy goat were ejected from the stadium and supposedly placed a curse on the team—and that explains the decades that have passed without another World Series appearance.

For some people the sense that events are both structured and connected is quite distorted. In 1958, the German psychiatrist Klaus Conrad coined the term *apophenia* for an "unmotivated seeing of connections" accompanied by a "specific experience of an abnormal meaningfulness." Apophenia is a well-recognized symptom of schizophrenia. When people with schizophrenia experience florid hallucinations, they have a tendency to interpret random events as not only meaningfully connected but often related to themselves, a tendency that forms the basis for paranoid delusions.

This propensity to detect co-occurrences and patterns lies at the heart of many supernatural assumptions. The neuropsychologist Peter Brugger of the University of Zurich recently proposed that this propensity stems from the relative activity of the neurotransmitter dopamine in the left and right cortical hemispheres of the brain. Brugger and his colleagues have consistently found that excessive dopamine activity in the right hemisphere is associated with apophenia and the assumption of supernatural forces.

To test his hypothesis, Brugger identified two groups of individuals—those who tended to believe in supernatural phenomena and those who were skeptics. To measure the study participants' sensitivity to patterns, Brugger administered a perception test using images of real faces, scrambled faces, real words, and non-words. Real faces and words have an identifiable pattern, but scrambled faces and non-words do not.

Study participants had to pick out the real words and faces as a series of images was flashed on a screen, too quickly for them to look at them carefully. As Brugger expected, the skeptics scored lower than the "believers;" they were more likely, for example, to call a real face a non-face. But after he administered L-dopa, a precursor to dopamine, to both groups, he found that the skeptics were significantly more likely to identify faces and words that previously they would have rejected as non-patterns.

Brugger believes that the activity of dopamine is related to the brain's ability to discriminate between meaningful signals and noise and that those individuals in whom this neurotransmitter system is overactive are more inclined to see causal connections and patterns. Though all people experience this inclination to some extent, it is elevated in psychiatric disorders such as schizophrenia and in temporarily distorted brain states resulting from the abuse of psychoactive drugs that affect the dopaminergic system, such as Ecstasy.

In *The Psychology of Superstition*, psychologist Gustav Jahoda argues that the conceptions we develop about our world are an integral part of human mental functioning that conferred a distinct survival advantage on our ancestors because they enable humans to exert some control over events. However, while science confines itself to observable events and readily jettisons a hypothesis that fails to account for all the facts, superstition focuses entirely on controlling the outcome of events. Evidence for the effectiveness of the control methods does not matter nearly as much as *belief* in the effectiveness of those methods.

We develop these conceptions from the moment we are born. By the age of two, for example, children have started to recognize that other people have minds and can initiate their own actions. They also understand that the thought of a dog is not the same as a real dog. By preschool they recognize that objects have volume and mass and fall when dropped, which suggests the existence of a force pulling things downward. In short, by a very young age children have developed reliable notions that include a grasp of the fact that wishes by themselves do not affect the physical world.

Many superstitions go beyond these notions, however. People who embrace a superstition believe implicitly that the mind can influence the physical world, or they attribute a theory of mind to inanimate objects. Psychologists Marjaana Lindeman and Kia Aarnio found that superstitious people were far more likely than skeptics to attribute mental abilities to water, furniture, and other material things. Tigers pitcher Mark "The Bird" Fidrych would relate. He would talk to the ball between pitches and ask the umpire to throw a ball back into the ball bag if it had been hit safely "so it would goof around with the other balls in there. Maybe it will learn some sense and come out as a pop-up next time."

Superstitions also attribute mysterious powers to physical objects. When a player refuses to wash his hat during a hitting streak, he's investing the object with powers that could be removed by soap and water. Bruce Hood tells of offering an audience $30 to put on a secondhand sweater. Everyone in the audience was willing—until Hood told them that a notorious murderer had once worn the sweater. Then all but one declined.

Psychologist Paul Rozin of the University of Pennsylvania has written about this belief in psychological contagion: the idea that a non-physical, usually negative state that we associate with the mind can transfer to objects. Rozin found that if people had developed a sense of revulsion toward certain things (such as feces, dirt, illness, disease, or putrefaction) in early childhood, they were later unwilling to touch objects that they believed to be contaminated by a disgusting item, even though the object had been thoroughly disinfected and cleaned. Rationality succumbed to these feelings: People even avoided objects that had never been in actual contact with a contaminant, such as a brand-new bedpan.

Recent brain imaging work suggests that superstitious feelings of disgust are difficult to control consciously. When Princeton psychologists Lasana Harris and Susan Fiske showed undergraduate students pictures of disgusting people and objects while the students lay in a functional magnetic resonance imaging scanner, they found that the images activated the amygdala and insula systems of the brain, which are associated with nausea.

What separates the superstitious from those who maintain mature, reliable notions about the world around them?

Lindeman and Aarnio devised an experiment to find out.

They used a questionnaire to identify students who were either strongly superstitious or strongly rational and had them take an online quiz. The superstitious people were far more likely to find truth in the following:

- *Mentalizing matter.* Subjects read statements such as, "Old furniture knows things about the past," and, "When summer is warm, flowers want to bloom." Then they rated each statement on a scale ranging from "purely metaphorical" to "literally true."
- *Physicalizing the mental.* Subjects were also asked to do the same with statements that applied physical properties to mental states, such as, "An unstable human mind is disintegrating."
- *Biologizing the mental.* Subjects assessed statements that misattributed biological properties to mental events, such as, "An evil thought is contaminated."

The authors also investigated the subjects' confusion between intentional and non-intentional events by telling them a story about a random, a natural, and a purposeful event, and then asking them to rate whether or not the outcome had a purpose. Superstitious people were more likely to say that natural phenomena such as storms happened for a reason. They also scored higher on measures of intuitive thinking and emotional instability than their more skeptical counterparts.

While no one has ever tested whether baseball players are more superstitious than average, Lindeman and Aarnio found that the average person is rather superstitious. But even highly rational people may embrace a superstition in times of crisis, especially when the stakes are high—when a loved one is seriously ill, for example, or a hurricane is approaching.

Giora Keinan, a professor at Tel Aviv University, found that among the 174 people who filled out questionnaires about the Iraqi Scud missile attacks during the 1991 Gulf War, those who reported the highest level of stress were most likely to endorse magical beliefs about entering a bomb shelter, such as, "I have the feeling that the chances of being hit during a missile attack are greater if a person whose house was attacked is present in the sealed room," and, "To be on the safe side, it is best to step into the sealed room right foot first."

Keinan noted that people who have these beliefs or practice such rituals often realize that they are not reasonable or rational but continue their behavior anyway. Stuart Vyse, a professor of psychology at Connecticut College, argues that such behavior may be harmless; in the case of Skinner's pigeons, the behavior at best allows the bird to eat and survive; at worst, the bird sacrifices nothing by turning in a circle or cocking its head. Other research has demonstrated how easy it is to elicit superstitious beliefs in people who consider themselves rational. Princeton University psychologist Emily Pronin has studied sports fans specifically and has spoken about practices such as crossing one's fingers and reciting a silent mantra when a basketball team's poorest free-throw shooter steps to the line—and then feeling gratified if he makes the free-throw.

Pronin based one experiment on her observation that spectators at sporting events seem to believe they can influence a team's performance mentally. Her subjects consisted of high school and college students who were told they were involved in an experiment to test spectators' influence on athletic performance. Each was asked to watch the performance of another member of the group selected to shoot free-throws blindfolded. The selection of the shooter was rigged so the same person would be chosen every time, and unbeknownst to the rest of the group, the shooter actually could see through the blindfold as he shot a toy basketball at a net.

Half of the spectators were instructed to try to influence the shooter's performance through "visualization," which consisted of thinking about each of eight statements provided in a packet—one for each shot. The other half were instructed to visualize the shooter lifting a dumbbell or engaging in some other random act. For both groups, the shooter was instructed to make about six of the eight shots.

Sure enough, those subjects who generated positive visualizations prior to successful shots felt more responsible for the shooter's success. Pronin and her coauthors say this finding helps explain why some fans are determined to watch their team play in a key game and remain in front of the television, rooting hard, at especially important moments. Wary of relaxing our support at such key times, we wait to grab another soda from the fridge or go to the bathroom.

Such thinking is the basis not only of the rituals and superstitions of sports fans, but also of voodoo and other activities intended to impose a curse on others. In the other experiment Pronin and her colleagues conducted, subjects stuck pins in a voodoo doll in an effort to cause physical pain to the person represented by the doll.

Pronin divided thirty-six subjects into two groups. One group included an obnoxious participant who arrived late, behaved rudely, and wore a T-shirt emblazoned with the slogan, "Stupid people shouldn't breed." When subjects were paired and asked to draw slips to determine who would be the "witch doctor" and who would be the "victim," the drawing was rigged so the obnoxious participant would always be the victim. In the other group, the person who played the obnoxious participant also was picked each time, but this time his behavior and appearance were ordinary. This was done to induce members of the first group to develop genuinely negative thoughts about the person playing the victim.

Before proceeding with the experiment, which involved sticking five pins into a doll with the victim's name pinned to it, each participant was given a moment to think about the subject—an act they were told would enhance the voodoo power. Presumably those who found the subject obnoxious would think ill of him, and these negative thoughts would make them feel more responsible when the victim feigned a headache as the "witch doctor" stuck pins into the doll. As expected, those who harbored negative thoughts about the victim were more likely than the others to believe that they really had caused the victim's headache.

Baseball fans will surely identify with the participants in these experiments. One of the pleasures of watching a game is the secret belief that cheering for the home team and thinking positive thoughts will somehow enhance their performance, while booing and wishing failure for opposing players will somehow cause them to lose.

ROOTING RELIGIOUSLY

Another angle on human superstition as it relates to sports fandom is to compare it with religion, which can be viewed as a form of superstition. (For a different take, see Chapter 7.) Pascal Boyer, a psychologist and anthropologist at Washington University in St. Louis, has suggested four explanations for religion that point to very deep human needs to understand experience, alleviate anxiety, and maintain social order:

- The human mind demands explanations.
- The human heart seeks comfort.
- Human society requires order.
- The human intellect is illusion-prone.

By now these explanations sound familiar. The first two, especially, resonate with why we might believe a team is cursed.

As Hood writes, "A belief in the supernatural can give people a deep sense of connection with the past and with each other. Such beliefs impart a consideration of the possibility that the mind will outlive the body."

Of course, superstitious beliefs also give sports fans a sense of connection with their team and with one another, and that, quite simply, is fun. Superstitions build solidarity among teammates as well as fans because they indicate a mutual desire for success. Superstitions indicate: "I really, *really* want my team to win." Nobody who cares about sports would call that irrational.

- 5 -

RISKS AND ASTERISKS
Neurological Enhancements in Baseball

BENNETT FODDY, PH.D.

The soul of sport is the enhancement of human athletic performance—through practice, through coaching, and through training. But the *story* of sport for the past three decades has been a story of performance enhancement using drugs.

In professional baseball, as in every other professional sport, the drug most often used to build muscle, boost power, and fuel scandal is the anabolic steroid. In 2001, Barry Bonds slugged a record 0.863 while allegedly using the designer steroid THG to improve his hitting power. Slugging percentage measures the total bases a player reaches divided by his number of at bats—a higher percentage suggests that a player often hits the ball a long way. Bonds took the record from Babe Ruth, who had held it for eighty-one years. And there are those who would like to put an asterisk next to this and other records Bonds has set, as though he had hit every ball with a tailwind.

But those who rush to attribute Bonds's success to steroid

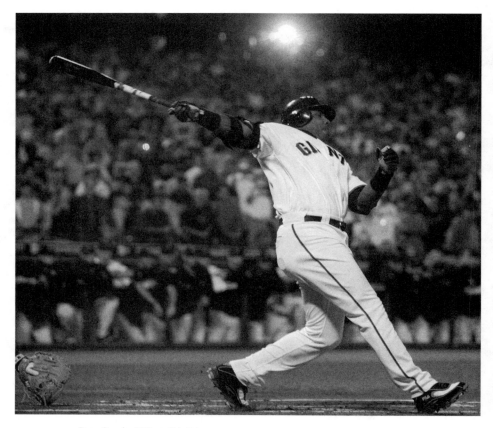

Barry Bonds. AP Photo/Eric Risberg.

use should consider this: Ruth cannot have been on steroids, and to look at his photos, he cannot have been anywhere near as strong as Bonds. In the end, a player's batting average, home run total, and slugging percentage all measure how *well* the ball is hit, not how muscular or strong the player is. To repeatedly hit the ball a long way, a player has to hit it accurately, no matter how much muscle goes into the swing.

What this example shows is that baseball is a sport in

which the usual set of performance enhancements is ill-suited to enhancing a player's numbers. The core skills of baseball—pitching, catching, and hitting—are not best enhanced by drugs that make a player stronger or faster. The strongest players can still miss the ball or hit it straight up in the air.

In fact, baseball—like golf, cricket, or archery—is a quintessentially brain-centered sport. The most important weapons any player has are in his brain: the speed of his reflexes, his spatial processing, his vision, and his fine-tuned muscle

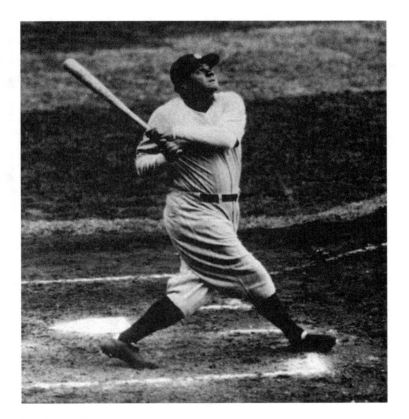

Babe Ruth. AP Photo

memory. In the case of baseball, only the ball needs to go faster, higher, and longer.

Of course, there are already enhancements that affect these neurological capacities—a group of drugs known as neurotropic (nerve-altering) drugs. For nearly every neurological disorder or disease, there is a pharmacological substance that addresses it. Most of these neurotropic substances are just as effective at modifying the functioning of a healthy athlete's brain. We have drugs that can alter a ballplayer's reflexes, mood, and cognitive processing. Drugs of abuse, too, are all neurotropic drugs.

Major League Baseball bans all drugs of abuse and since 2006 has banned a few neurotropic substances. That means that players could be, and likely are, using neurotropic drugs to enhance their performance today. In fact, although Senator George Mitchell's report in 2007 on drug use in professional baseball was limited to prohibited strength enhancers such as steroids and growth hormone, Mitchell acknowledged the rumored use of neurotropic drugs.

WHAT'S AVAILABLE?

Neurological enhancement sounds far-fetched, like something from a science-fiction novel. But human beings have long been ingesting substances that improve their neurological functions. At the 1972 Summer Olympics, soon after drug testing had begun in earnest, every athlete who was caught doping was using a stimulant such as amphetamine or ephedrine. Even in the original Olympic marathons of ancient Greece, the marathon runners would use strychnine as a stimulant.

Stimulants are perhaps the most obvious type of neurological enhancement that could be used in a skill-based sport such

78

as baseball. Stimulants, broadly, increase activity in the brain by increasing the availability of neurotransmitters, which in turn increase the rate of the brain's functioning as well as other neurologically mediated functions such as heart rate.

For a ballplayer, one of the most useful effects of a stimulant is that it can reduce the time it takes for him to read and react to a pitch. As John Milton and his colleagues point out in this volume (see Chapter 3), it can take a batter almost as much time to respond to a pitch as it does for the ball to travel to the plate. The batter tries to anticipate the trajectory of the ball based on the body movement of the pitcher, but in many cases he has little or no time to make decisions between the moment he sees the pitch and the moment he swings the bat. If a stimulant can shave mere milliseconds off a player's reaction times, this decision interval could be substantially increased.

A variety of drugs could fit the bill. Cocaine is a stimulant with a long history of sporting use. In the 1890s, while it was still popular for its medicinal properties, cocaine was given to professional cyclists toward the end of a race to relieve fatigue. As an enhancement, it would be much more effective in modern baseball. Apart from elevating a player's mood and confidence levels, it would speed up his reflexes; researchers Robert Hienz and colleagues found that it shortens the reaction time of baboons by 10 percent.

Amphetamines produce little or no enhancement in reaction time but significantly reduce the effect of fatigue on a person's ability to track a moving object such as a ball. Dextroamphetamine, an amphetamine variant that is popular as a recreational drug, improves decision-making and reduces impulsivity in healthy human beings, which would be an effective enhancement for batters who tend to swing at balls outside the strike zone.

Major league players are already using amphetamines to improve their reflexes, and a number have been caught using cocaine. While the full extent of stimulant use is not known, it is rumored to be extremely widespread. At the infamous Pittsburgh trials of 1985, Cardinals first baseman Keith Hernandez admitted using cocaine and suggested that 40 percent of major league players were using the drug.

Amphetamine use is rumored to be even more widespread. Former player Tony Gwynn told the *New York Times* in 2003 that amphetamine use was rife in the professional game: "People might think there is a steroid problem in baseball, but it's nowhere near the other problem; the other, it's a rampant problem. . . . Guys feel like steroids are cheating and greenies [amphetamines] aren't." In his 1969 tour diary, Yankees pitcher Jim Bouton quotes a teammate as saying this about amphetamine use: "Just about the whole Baltimore team takes them. Most of the Tigers. Most of the guys on this club. And that's just what I know for sure."

Amphetamines and cocaine are on baseball's banned list under the banner of "drugs of abuse," but illegal drugs aren't the only effective way of reducing a player's reaction time. A number of other stimulants are available, some of which are banned in international athletics and some of which are not. From methylphenidate (Ritalin) to caffeine, there is a very wide range of substances available, by prescription or over the counter, that may reduce a person's reaction time to some extent.

The attitude toward prescription drugs in American culture has changed dramatically during the past century. Initially, significant amounts of cocaine were included in Coca-Cola. Until 1941, amphetamines could be bought without a prescription. The last twenty years has seen a marked rise in the prescription of stimulants and in the consumption of those that, like caffeine, occur in foods. There is no bright line between any of these stimulants—caffeine and Ritalin are habit-forming like amphetamines and can produce similar side effects from acute or prolonged overuse.

The traditional stimulants produce unwanted side effects that could reduce a player's performance, such as tremor or anxiety. But there are newer stimulants available that clearly reduce reaction time without producing the unwanted side effects. One example is the class of drugs known as ampakines, which includes a popular drug called modafinil.

Modafinil, prescribed to treat narcolepsy and on baseball's banned list since 2006, has been found to improve not only reaction time but pattern recognitition, working memory, and spatial planning. Players on modafinil might well be able to detect the ball earlier, figure out where it is headed sooner, and be better at stopping themselves from swinging at balls outside the strike zone. In rats, it reduces reaction time by around 25 percent; if it were even one-tenth as effective in humans, modafinil would provide a large competitive advantage. Athletes have already been caught using it as a doping agent in international athletics competitions.

Stimulants may be the most widely used neurological enhancements, but they are not the only ones available. As Milton and his colleagues point out, the process of hitting a ball with a bat depends on a number of distinct neurological processes. The batter tries to anticipate the trajectory of the ball before it is pitched, from the action of the pitcher. He tries to pick out the ball in flight and estimate when and where it will arrive over the plate. He tries to take into account where all the fielders are and whether there are men on base. To be a baseball genius, you don't need a college education, yet it seems reasonable to suggest that drugs that improve a player's cognitive abilities would improve his ability to hit the ball over the fence.

Drugs that would help a player to perform these mental gymnastics already exist. Drugs known as nootropics, or "smart drugs," increase the amount of a neurotransmitter in the brain called acetylcholine, increasing the brain's metabolic rate. It is thought that these drugs improve a person's memory and ability to focus and make calculations, among other things. The effects of existing nootropic drugs are mild, and there is no clear consensus on whether or why they work; one of the better known, Piracetam, is not even banned by the World Anti-Doping Agency (WADA). But the gap in performance between professional ballplayers is slim, and performance-enhancing effects that would be therapeutically useless could still make a noticeable competitive difference. In the near future, there may be more-effective nootropic drugs that confer a more substantial advantage.

Finally, there are drugs that offer relief for the negative symptoms that come from playing the big game. When a game is close, or when the stakes are high, the players become nervous. In the worst cases, they "choke," producing a performance well below their ability. To succeed at the highest level, a baseball player must shut out his emotions, the visual distractions in the grandstand, and his doubts.

The effects of stage fright are not merely emotional or psychological. With the bases loaded and the score tied in the bottom of the ninth, a ballplayer's heart rate increases. He may suffer nausea, shallow breath, and, critically, reduced muscular control. He trembles or stumbles. He sweats and drops the ball through slippery fingers. This loss of physical competence makes stage fright a self-fulfilling fear. Professional violinists or pianists frequently try to break this cycle by using the beta-blocker class of drugs. Beta-blockers essentially inhibit the ability of adrenaline to stimulate the beta receptors in the organs of the body. This reduces the physiological symptoms of stage fright—it causes the muscles to relax and the heart rate to become steadier. In sports that require competitors to remain calm and skillful rather than explosively athletic, this confers a huge advantage. Beta-blockers are banned in competitive international billiards, gymnastics, and archery, but not in Major League Baseball.

Even with symptomatic relief for stage fright, the emotions of a high-pressure game can still damage a player's performance. A study by Alexander J. Shackman and colleagues found that when subjects were made anxious by being repeatedly startled, they performed much worse at spatial tasks. Baseball is nothing if not a spatial task—if a person could be made less anxious using anxiety-reducing drugs (such as Valium), antidepressants, or even recreational drugs, he would likely perform better at the spatial calculations involved in throwing balls and swinging bats, at least in high-stakes, high-pressure games.

One drug that could reduce the psychological impact of a high-stress sporting situation is cannabis. Cannabis is well known for impairing motor skills and concentration, and yet many players who have been caught with the drug in their blood have been at the top of sports that stress agility, skill, and spatial processing in the same manner as baseball. Ross Regabliati won the Olympic gold medal for snowboarding in 1998 before testing positive for marijuana use. Baseball players—especially the anxious ones—could use it to their advantage.

If that seems outlandish, consider this: Dock Ellis claims he pitched a no-hitter for the Pittsburgh Pirates in 1970 while high on LSD. LSD would normally be considered an impediment to spatial and perceptual tasks, and as Ellis told interviewers many years later: "The ball was small sometimes, the ball was large sometimes, sometimes I saw the catcher, sometimes I didn't."

In studying golfers putting, Sian Beilock and Thomas Carr found that one of the major causes of choking was *attending to proceduralized skills.* If you think about what you should be doing, rather than just doing it, your performance suffers. Perhaps this explains why Ellis's hallucinations did not stand in the way of a no-hitter; he performed the task with his fine-tuned muscle skills unhindered by self-conscious thought.

There is a smorgasbord of neurological enhancements available to the professional baseball player today. As time goes on, more will become available. Neurotropic drugs such as nootropics and anxiety-reducing anxiolytics are in heavy demand, and billions of dollars are being spent each year in the search for new drugs. If the rumors are to be believed, baseball has been a sport of pharmaceutical neuroenhancement for decades, and the trend will almost certainly continue as newer, better neurological enhancements are invented.

Of the neurotropic drugs available today, only a tiny proportion are currently illegal in the major leagues, which means that we can reasonably assume that many professional ball-players use some kind of neurological enhancement. Some of these enhancements, including amphetamines and ana-bolic steroids, have negative side effects. Others, such as beta-blockers, caffeine, and modafinil, seem to be entirely safe at effective doses. Should we care if neurological enhancement becomes the norm in the professional game?

WHAT'S GOOD

In sport worldwide, there is an almost universal presumption that it is worth prohibiting the use of performance-enhanc-ing drugs, and that it is worth spending a great deal of money enforcing the bans. WADA, which governs drug testing in most international sports, budgeted almost $26 million for its 2007 activities. This money, which comes from govern-ments around the world as well as from the Olympic move-ment, underlines the importance societies worldwide give to the drug bans.

Major League Baseball, meanwhile, permits players to use a range of effective neurotropic enhancements that are banned by WADA. In this sense, baseball is out of step with the international anti-doping movement. Who is right: the major leagues, or the world anti-doping regulator? To answer this, we need to be able to explain why doping regulations are important.

WADA writes the rules that govern drug use in interna-tional sport, and its rulebook gives an explicit rationale for the ban on performance-enhancing drugs:

> Anti-doping programs seek to preserve what is intrinsically valu-able about sport. This intrinsic value is often referred to as "the

spirit of sport"; it is the essence of Olympism; it is how we play true. The spirit of sport is the celebration of the human spirit, body and mind. . . . Doping is fundamentally contrary to the spirit of sport.

Unfortunately, WADA never explains why doping is contrary to this "celebration of the human spirit, body and mind," and it never explains why sport's value depends on this "celebration." It begs the question: Why is it that a player can "play true" on dietary supplements such as creatine, but not on hormones such as steroids? Why can a player celebrate the human spirit on caffeine, but not on amphetamines? (For another take on these questions, see the sidebar on page 87.)

WADA's rather ambiguous explanation of the need for drug testing is emblematic of a debate that has been dominated by gut feelings, vague generalizations, and moral panic. But to make accurate ethical judgments about drugs and drug testing, we only need to weigh up what is good or bad about performance-enhancing drugs and what is good or bad about the process of enforcing anti-doping rules.

In any sport, new rules are usually introduced with at least one of two groups in mind: the players and the spectators. In 1971, helmets were introduced in the major leagues to improve occupational safety for players, without reducing the enjoyment of fans. In contrast, the strike zone has been reduced twice since 1969 in order to increase the number of hits, which makes things more interesting for the fans but not for the players.

Sometimes, a technology or method of training appears that is good for both the players *and* the fans. In baseball, ironically, the best example of such a win-win technology is the one class of drug that is currently banned in the major leagues—anabolic steroids.

Winning, Cheating Have Ancient Roots

The Washington Post   *August 3, 2007*

By Sally Jenkins

Maybe we shouldn't ask athletes to live up to ideals that, let's face it, are unsupported by the chronically weak performance of human nature. Maybe it's time to decriminalize performance-enhancing drugs, in view of the fact that the first drug cheat was an ancient Greek and runners brought sport-doping into the modern age in 1904 by dosing themselves with strychnine.

Our Air Force gives fighter jocks "go-pills" to get them through long missions, but we don't refuse to call them heroes because they're on speed. So what's this strange amnesia that causes us to seek purity in athletes? Why should they have to meet a higher moral standard than soldiers? Call me naive.

Many of us are cringing at the prospect that Barry Bonds will break Hank Aaron's home run record, starting with yours truly, because of allegations he used performance enhancers. A record should be joyful, but this one makes us regretful. Why should Bonds's personal health choices matter to us so much? Because he forces us to address head-on the possibility that sports have become utterly riddled with doping. If so, then legalizing performance enhancers may be the most honest thing we could do. But it doesn't make anyone happy to say so.

What's the job of an athlete, really? It is to seek the limits of the human body, for our viewing pleasure. Athletes are astronauts of the physique, explorers. Some of them choose to explore by making human guinea pigs out of themselves. So maybe we should quit assigning any ethical value to what they do, and simply enjoy their feats as performance artists. Virtue was another notion dreamed up by the Greeks, only they were a lot less confused about what they meant by the term. Their word for virtue could also be accurately translated as simply "excellence." As for the word "amateur," it didn't exist to them at all.

The ancient Olympic champions were professionals who competed for huge cash prizes as well as olive wreaths, lived on the public dole and were sometimes recruited by competing cities seeking status. Most forms of what we would call cheating were perfectly acceptable to them, save for game-fixing. There is evidence that they gorged themselves on meat—not a normal dietary staple of the Greeks—and experimented with herbal medications in an effort to enhance their performances. Olympic scholar William Blake Tyrell, author of "The Smell of Sweat: Greek Athletics, Olympics, and Culture," has observed: "Winning was everything. If they thought a rhinoceros horn would help them win, they would have ground it up."

According to Charles Yesalis, professor of health and human development at

Penn State and a longtime scholar of performance enhancement, the ancient Greek athletes also drank wine potions, used hallucinogens and ate animal hearts or testicles in search of potency. "We've never had clean sport," he says.

Doping is not a modern art. It's just the medicine that's new. As a recent story in *National Geographic* pointed out, performance enhancement grew with chemistry in the mid-19th century. Athletes choked down sugar cubes dipped in ether, brandy laced with cocaine, nitroglycerine and amphetamines. In that context, the current scourges of steroids and blood boosters are merely a sequential progression.

Opponents of legalizing performance enhancers argue against it on two main grounds: 1) it would open up a doping arms race in which athletes who could afford the best drugs would have an unfair advantage, and 2) doping is injurious to the health of the athletes. But the arms race is already on—and it has been for centuries. That genie is out of the bottle, and there's no putting it back. As for the ill effects of performance enhancers, there is a very strong argument to be made that legalization would actually help in risk reduction, make it easier to control the types of risks athletes are taking.

Furthermore, it's impossible to draw the line any more between what is an artificial enhancement and what is a natural one. Is there a real difference between voluntary LASIK eye surgery, a small controlled dose of testosterone or EPO, or sleeping in an altitude tent that produces the same effect as EPO, only without the needle?

The next step in the sequential progression is gene therapy—athletes will be able to inject genes that build muscle. At which point steroids will seem as crude as sugar cubes soaked in ether.

The stark truth is that great athletes are fundamentally very different from you and me. They are freaks of nature, with uncanny hand-eye coordination or peripheral vision randomly assigned in the gene pool. They can seem nearly a different species. And they are quite often profoundly cold elitists whose moral code is different from ours, too. To many of them, the performance is all and what they find unnatural is to leave some physical possibility untapped. "They're highly paid entertainers, and they get paid to win and that's what they're trying to do," Yesalis says.

In an odd way, legalizing performance enhancers might restore some candor to what we're watching. It would end a charade and help us sort out truly criminal behavior from that which merely offends our idealism. But personally, every time I come to that conclusion, I find myself backing away from it, reluctant to say it's the definitive answer.

The price of legalization is that we give up our ideals about athletes once and for all, and that's a painful prospect. We gave up our ideals about actors, singers and politicians and various other kinds of professionals a long time ago, but that doesn't mean we enjoyed doing it. "If there was drug available for journalists, professors or lawyers, they would take it," Yesalis theorizes. "Why do you think it would be just athletes?" That's true. But it's a sorry fact.

Legalization is not likely to happen, because most of us prefer illusion to reality. Games are stories we tell ourselves, and as such, we seem to need some moral content in them, as opposed to the capricious traumas, sad erosions and ambiguities of everyday reality. Yesalis likens performance enhancers to the special effects in a film.

"When you go to a movie, you don't want to see how the movie was made, or the special effects are done," he says. "The drama plays out and it has a black or white ending. You just want to be entertained and happy or sad your team won [or lost]."

Steroids can make a batter run faster or make a pitcher throw the ball faster. But they also can aid players in recovering from injury and training. This recuperative use of steroids was a major focus of the 2002 investigation that led to the introduction of drug testing. The Florida Marlins' Chad Fox said to Barry Bloom of the official Major League Baseball Web site: "With all the injuries I've had, I could have taken steroids. But my family is too important."

When he made this statement, Fox was referring to the period before testing began, so he could not have meant that his family would suffer if he was banned for doping. He meant that his family would be put at grave risk by the side effects steroids would have on his body. But when taken in clinical doses, anabolic steroids are a safe and effective method for reducing recuperation time after sporting injuries. In order to elicit both the muscle-building effects of steroids and their famous health-endangering side effects, an athlete must take very large quantities.

If Fox had taken the steroids in modest doses, it would only have lengthened his career and helped him to recover from injuries, which would have been good for the fans, for Fox, and certainly for his family.

When changes occur in a sport, they are rarely as all-around good as steroids are for baseball. What makes a sport good for players, such as safety and good sportsmanship, often makes things worse for spectators. And the things that make a sport more attractive to fans, such as night games and television cameras, often make things worse for the players.

Sporting bodies, pundits, and players often talk about what's good for their sport. Drugs are often said to be bad for a sport. But that is an oversimplification. Drugs can be good for players and bad for fans, or vice versa. In fact, whether the drug is good for the fans or for the players depends on what kind of drug it is.

NEUROENHANCEMENTS FROM THE FAN'S PERSPECTIVE

Neurological enhancements, many of which are legal in baseball, do not help players to recuperate like steroids do. To assess whether a particular drug is good or bad from a spectator's point of view, we need to know where the value lies for the spectator. What's good about watching a game of baseball?

In the first place, any spectator sport is valued by fans as a source of entertainment. To this end, the sport must be dramatic—it needs to put the players in situations that are tense or emotional, and it needs to generate sympathetic excitement in the onlookers. Anxiety-reducing drugs such as cannabis or Valium would prevent choking and lower players' stress but diminish the entertainment enormously. Imagine the game of baseball without the chokes, without the dummy spits, without the stage fright. These are neurological phenomena, which can be "cured" using neurological enhancements. But they are also the source of much of the game's drama.

By contrast, if players used stimulants to improve their reaction times, the effect would be more or less invisible to spectators. In fact, the long-term use of traditional stimulants such as amphetamines or caffeine tends to increase anxiety and even aggression, which would heighten the emotionality of players and produce more dramatic confrontations. From a fan's point of view, the best games might be those in which all the players are hyperactive, anxious, aggressive, and unstable.

Of course, baseball is also a game of history, statistics, and record-keeping. Perhaps because it's less athletic than football or hockey, the statistics are more important and more interesting, and the records stand for a longer period of time. Babe Ruth's career home run record lasted thirty-nine years; then the record was held by Hank Aaron from 1974 to 2007. These records withstood years of rule changes, equipment development, and the end of segregation. Few games have records that are as meaningful and robust as the records in baseball, and that is part of the game's appeal for fans. If players using neurotropic drugs performed noticeably better than the players of old, the old records and achievements would quickly lose their importance.

But hold on. Dock Ellis was pitching on LSD in 1970. Amphetamines were invented more than a century ago and were not made illegal until 1986. Hank Aaron admits he used them during the 1960s. There is no reason to suggest that the use of amphetamines or other enhancements in professional baseball is a recent trend. When Major League Baseball began screening for drugs of abuse in 2003, players such as Barry Bonds were denied enhancements that were freely available to the likes of Aaron. From a record-keeping perspective, the best thing would be to ban modern, safe enhancements such as modafinil and permit players to use the more harmful, old-fashioned enhancements that were used by some of the all-time greats.

NEUROENHANCEMENTS FROM THE PLAYER'S PERSPECTIVE

When a drug appears that confers a massive performance benefit but no ill health effects, it cannot be bad for baseball players. In international athletics, poorer players are frequently disadvantaged by the existence of drugs and training methods that are only accessible to the rich. In Major League Baseball, there *are* no poor players. If everyone needs to take a new drug to stay competitive, and that drug is safe, then the players are not made any worse off than if a new brand of shoe is introduced or a new sporting diet is concocted. Modafinil, for example, would cheaply enhance players' performance without causing side effects much worse than a headache.

When a drug appears that confers both dose-dependent performance benefits and dose-dependent health consequences, it puts the players in a double bind. If every batter on every team were taking high doses of a harmful drug, the players would be forced to make a choice between remaining competitive and protecting their health. It is better for players if drugs such as these are never invented. That is the reason that steroids are a problem in strength-based sports: the higher the dose, the stronger the athlete. This provides an incentive to take unreasonably large doses of steroids. But higher doses also carry higher risks.

However, most of the available neurological enhancements do not share this strength incentive without limit. Amphetamines, cocaine, and caffeine enhance skillful performance up to a point, but extremely high doses intoxicate a player or even kill him. To remain competitive, a ballplayer might have to take *some* stimulants, but not a massive, life-endangering dose.

Nevertheless, the use of stimulants cannot be said to be a *good* thing from the players' perspective. In the best-case scenario, everyone takes a safe dose of a drug, so that no unfair advantage is granted to players who dope. But if every player took stimulants, then everyone's reaction times would improve, and nobody would get any kind of advantage.

If every player used stimulants, there would be no competitive advantage, but that does not mean that the players' experience would go unchanged. During the game, their brains would become charged with dopamine and adrenaline, creating a feeling of euphoria, a tensing of the muscles, and a thumping heart. After the game they might have sleepless nights or find themselves seeking more of the drug, as an in-game habit turned into an off-field dependency. As time went by, as their brains adapted to regular doses of the stimulants, they would become anxious and aggressive. Using traditional stimulants over a long period, a player's brain would change in ways that would make the game—and life—worse for him.

By contrast, sedatives, euphorics, anxiolytics, and beta-blockers might improve a player's enjoyment of the game by relieving anxiety and stage fright, reducing heart rate, and decreasing the activation of the brain's neurons. Players could relax their muscles and their brains and swing the bat as comfortably as they would in the practice cage. As I pointed out above, this would be bad news for the fans.

So the drugs that are good for the players are not the drugs that are good for the fans. To complicate matters, the drug-testing process is itself bad for fans *and* players. It is bad for the fans because it raises ticket prices, casts doubt on superstars, and overshadows the game. And it is bad for the players because they must endure invasive tests and constant suspicion.

WHO MATTERS MORE?

The fact that the neurological enhancements that would be acceptable to the fans are not the same ones that should be acceptable to players creates a conflict that neurological science cannot solve for us. Who is more important: the fans or the players? Whose needs should be given priority?

Historically, a kind of uneasy balance has been struck between the interests of the spectators and those of major league ballplayers. For example, there is a relationship that links the wages paid to players and the amount that fans and TV networks must pay to see the game. Whenever wages threaten to fall too low, the players will go on strike, as they did in 1994. At the same time, if admission prices rise too much, or if TV licensing deals become too expensive for the networks, the spectators will stop watching.

If we were to give priority to the needs of baseball players, we would allow them to take sedatives, antidepressants, or beta-blockers to overcome the stress of the major leagues. We would allow injured players to use steroids to recover more quickly.

If we wished to give precedence to the fans' needs, and maximize ticket revenues, then we would give the players intoxicating drugs such as alcohol to heighten emotion and widen the gap between the ice men and the chokers. We would try to make sure that factors such as spatial processing and vigilance remain at historic levels by permitting amphetamines and cocaine but banning safe new stimulants such as modafinil.

A broad-based ban of neurological enhancements would be equitable in the sense that it would be equally bad for all parties. It would be expensive, driving ticket prices up and player wages down. It would force players to choose between remaining competitive and remaining legal. It would inevitably result in the exclusion of popular players from the game, and it would overshadow the sport in scandal. It would be the worst of all possible options.

And yet, we should not be surprised if we soon see such a ban. International baseball already makes use of the all-inclusive WADA list of banned substances, as do other, similar skill-based sports, such as cricket, archery, and even chess. Major League Baseball has thus far resisted this ban everything approach, but the pressure to conform is mounting.

ENHANCING THE FANS

There is a neurological enhancement that can be prescribed to the fans instead of the players, to improve the neurological processes that constitute enjoyment of the game.

This neuroenhancement excites the brain's inhibitory GABA neurotransmitters and inhibits the excitatory glutamate neurotransmitters. It also causes a release of dopamine and serotonin in the brain's reward centers. As a result, it produces feelings of well-being and euphoria and encourages social participation in the spectatorship of the game.

Though there are severe side effects resulting from long-term use, including liver damage, cancer, and dependence, the medical consensus is that it can be used in moderate doses for its properties as an enhancement without creating an undue level of risk.

Happily, diluted, medical-strength beer is already sold at every major league venue.

– 6 –

BASEBALL AND HANDEDNESS

KENNETH M. HEILMAN, M.D.

Children learn at a very young age that they prefer to use one hand over the other and that not everyone prefers the same hand. When I started playing catch with my father I noted that I was throwing the ball with my right hand and he was throwing with his left.

Very often I would also play catch with my brother Fred, who preferred to throw the ball with his right hand but also could throw the ball very well with his left. Because my older brother was a good athlete, I thought I should learn to throw with either hand. But whenever I tried to throw with my left hand my brother would yell, "Kenny, throw with your right hand. You look terrible throwing with your left."

He was correct. Not only did it look terrible when I tried to throw with my left arm, but I could not throw as far, as fast, or as accurately as I did with my right hand.

At the time, I was not thinking about whether my brain had

something to do with my preference for throwing right-handed (and inability to throw with my left). I was far more concerned with how my Brooklyn Dodgers were doing. One of my favorite players on the Dodgers was Jackie Robinson. In addition to initiating integration, he helped the Dodgers win several National League pennants and finally beat the Bronx Bombers—the New York Yankees—in the 1955 World Series. Robinson, like me, was a right-hander, but I noticed that many of the greatest hitters batted left-handed. When my brother and father taught me to bat, they knew that I was right-handed and taught me to stand with my left shoulder forward, my right hand above my left, and the bat resting over my right shoulder.

But with the knowledge of all the great hitters who batted left-handed with their right shoulder forward and their left hand above their right, I decided I would practice batting like a lefty. When I learned to bat right-handed it immediately felt comfortable to hold the bat as described above, but when I tried to bat left-handed it felt uncomfortable. My swing was clumsy and I had trouble meeting the ball. As much as I tried I could never acquire the ability to bat left-handed.

I knew very little about the brain at this time, but I remained curious about why I could not bat or throw left-handed. I tried to nurture this batting skill but failed. Did nature prevail over nurture? While my love for the Dodgers and Major League Baseball ended when Walter O'Malley abandoned his loyal fans and moved the Dodgers to Los Angeles, my interest in handedness—and, with time, the role of the brain—has persisted.

In 1982, John McLean and Francis Ciurczak wrote a letter to the *New England Journal of Medicine* describing their study of handedness among Major League Baseball players (excluding pitchers). They divided their subjects into those who threw right-handed and batted right-handed (R/R), those who threw right-handed and batted left-handed (R/L), and those who both threw and batted left-handed (L/L). They found a higher percentage of left-handers (L/L) in the major leagues than in the general population. They also selected the forty-one best major league hitters of all time and found even a higher percentage of left-handed players (L/L) in this group than in either the general population or all players in the major leagues during the 1980 season.

The higher proportion of left-handed players in pro base-ball cannot be explained by an advantage in playing certain positions. There is no advantage to being right- or left-handed when playing the outfield. A left-handed first baseman has a better tagging angle on pick-off moves, but left-handed third basemen, shortstops, or second basemen are at a disadvantage because first base is to the left of these players and it is eas-ier to throw across one's body. In addition, most catchers are right-handed, probably because a left-handed catcher would have more problems throwing around the right-handed bat-ter when attempting to pick off a base runner attempting to steal second.

Several theories have attempted to account for the supe-riority of left-handed batters. One of them notes that a left-handed batter is closer to first base than is the right-handed hitter. In addition, when right-handed batters finish their swing they are facing third base and momentum is moving their bodies in that direction, while left-handed batters finish their swing facing and following through toward first base. These differences give left-handed batters an advantage in rapidly getting to first base.

Another theory suggests that left-handed batters are better able to see the windup and delivery of a right-handed pitcher, and most pitchers are right-handed. That would give lefties an advantage over right-handed hitters.

Neither of these ideas is supported by McLean and Ciurczak's analyses. They found that the L/L hitters had higher batting averages than the R/L hitters, who fared no better than the R/R hitters. If observing the pitcher, facing first base at the end of the swing, and gaining a step toward first base explained the superiority of those who bat left-handed, the group that throws right-handed but bats lefty (R/L) should match the L/L group, who both throw and bat left-handed, and each of these groups should be superior to the right-handed hitters. These observations suggest that my batting average may not have risen even if I had learned to bat left-handed—and that there is another reason for the superiority of the L/L hitters.

HAND PREFERENCE AND THE BRAIN

There are many theories about the origins of handedness, but most investigators now believe that hand preference is most likely related to asymmetries between the right and left sides of the brain. Clues as to why left-handed batters tend to be better than right-handed hitters may emerge from exploring how brain organization influences hand preference.

The first person to suggest that differences between the brain's hemispheres might account for handedness was Paul Broca. In 1865 he reported on eight right-handed patients who developed an impaired ability to speak and weakness of the right arm following brain injuries, such as a stroke, to one of their hemispheres. Because each hemisphere of the brain controls the opposite arm, Broca deduced that his patients' right-side weakness meant they had suffered injury to their left hemispheres. The loss of speech together with right-arm weakness suggested to Broca that hand preference might be related to which side of the brain mediates or programs speech and language, but he did not delve into this relationship.

The reason why the left hemisphere of right-handed people mediates speech and language remained unknown for more than 100 years, until Norman Geschwind and Walter Levitsky demonstrated in 1968 that humans have anatomic differences between the left and right hemispheres. Each of the senses has an area in the brain called the primary sensory cortex, where information is received. These sensory-receiving areas then send this information to an adjacent area of the brain called the sensory association cortex, which further processes the information that this sensory system is carrying into the brain.

Geschwind and Levitsky found that part of the auditory association cortex was often larger in the left hemisphere than in the right. Anatomists call this larger portion of the auditory association cortex the planum temporale (PT) and clinicians call this region of the brain Wernicke's area, after the neurologist who first noted that patients with damage to this area could not understand speech.

Geschwind and Levitsky's classic study was performed in patients who had died, and their handedness was not known. Thus, to learn more about the relationships between hand preference, language, and anatomic asymmetries of the brain hemispheres, our research group, led by Anne Foundas, measured the planum temporale in patients who had undergone selective hemispheric anesthesia, where one hemisphere is temporarily put to sleep, to determine their language laterality. We found that all eleven of our right-handed subjects lost their ability to speak when their left hemisphere was put to sleep, and all these patients had a larger PT in the left hemisphere. Unfortunately, we were able to test only one subject who was left-handed. Although a single subject is inconclusive, this subject was unable to speak when the right hemisphere was under anesthesia and had a larger planum temporale on the right side than on the left.

Although this study supports the hypothesis that the umpire's ability to literally call a batter out on strikes may come from the same hemisphere that determines with which hand he prefers to signal "You're out," the reason language's home in the brain would determine hand preference is unclear. It would seem that this preference might be related to communicative gestures and writing: Because in almost all right-handed people the left hemisphere mediates language and also controls the right hand, writing would give the left hemisphere direct access to the right hand but only indirect access to the left. Contradicting this theory, however, is the fact that most people are right-handed, even in cultures where many people have never learned to read and write. In addition, children show hand preference even before they learn to write. Many right-handed people who have language mediated by their left hemisphere prefer to gesture with their left hand. Finally, it is unclear why the hand that writes better would also be superior at throwing a ball or determining how a person would hold a bat. Thus, right-handedness in most people cannot be fully explained by a preference to use the right hand when writing or gesturing.

We often use our hands to alter the environment in pursuit of a goal or intention, and it is possible that language and verbal reasoning are the major source of intentions. One way we have learned about the relationships between language, intentions, and hand movement is by studying people with epilepsy. Sometimes an epileptic seizure can start on one side of the brain and progress to the other. When these types of seizures cannot be controlled by medications, their spread can be stopped by cutting the large cable, called the corpus callosum, that connects the two hemispheres. Studies of patients who had their corpus callosum cut to control seizures found that these patients are impaired in performing tasks where the two hemispheres must communicate.

These patients often experience what is called an alien hand. A patient of mine told me of an episode when she had put on a blue dress. She went to her closet to obtain some matching blue shoes, but when she picked them up with her right hand, her left hand grabbed the shoes out of her right hand, put them on the floor and picked up a red pair. The ensuing hand-to-hand combat ended with her left hand slamming the closet door on her right.

This and many similar stories suggest that the thoughts such patients are consciously aware of are the thoughts and desires of the language-dominant hemisphere. These patients are unaware of the thoughts and desires of the other hemisphere and consider the actions it mediates to be "alien." Based on these observations, it is possible that people with left-hemisphere language dominance, even in the presence of an intact corpus callosum, might prefer to use their right hand because this hand receives direct instructions from the left hemisphere and thus might be better able to carry out one's intentions and conscious goals.

Although language laterality might have some influence on hand preference, especially when hand-arm control is being influenced by verbal language, there is a weakness with both of these language-dominance hypotheses of handedness. In 1975, Theodore Rasmussen and Brenda Milner used selective hemisphere anesthesia to show that 70 percent of left-handed people had speech mediated by their left hemispheres, 15 percent had speech control in the right hemisphere, and the remaining 15 percent had bilateral hemispheric control of speech. Because this and subsequent studies have demonstrated that the majority of left-handed people have left-hemisphere language dominance, it is unlikely that language dominance alone can account for hand preference.

MOVEMENT MEMORIES

Carl Furillo, the great Brooklyn Dodgers outfielder, was known for throwing runners out at home plate from right field. His arm was so accurate and strong he was called the "Reading Rifle." In order for his throws to be that accurate, his brain had to program the muscles in the arm so that they made accurate movements with precise timing. Right-handed patients with corpus callosum injuries that interrupt the connection between the right and left hemispheres have been studied to see how they perform skilled tasks, such as showing the movements required to throw a ball or use a hammer. When attempting to perform these movements in response to verbal command, these patients perform well with their right hand but poorly with their left. In fact, their performance with their left hand is much worse than that of normal people attempting to perform these same tasks with their left arm and hand; sometimes these patients' left-handed attempts at performing skilled actions are so poor that the goals of these movements are difficult to recognize. The language-dominance hypothesis of handedness would suggest that their injury could have hindered them by disconnecting language areas in the left hemisphere from motor areas in the right hemisphere that control movements of the left hand.

But these patients' difficulties went beyond language; they also failed to imitate movements made by the examiner, and when given actual objects such as a hammer, they failed to use them properly. The ability to imitate movements and use actual objects does not require language. Because these patients could not correctly do either, researchers suggested that the left hemisphere not only mediates language but also controls the programming of purposeful skilled movements.

Hugo Liepmann, the first physician to systematically study the control of skilled movement in patients with neurological diseases, suggested in 1920 that hand preference could be attributed to what he called the *hemispheric laterality of movement* formula, or what today are called movement representations. Each hemisphere primarily controls the opposite, or contralateral, hand. According to Liepmann's model, when a person is attempting to perform a learned, skilled act with his preferred hand, the portions of the motor system that control the muscles of this hand (the opposite motor cortex) would have direct access to the movement knowledge that is stored in this same hemisphere. In contrast, the non-preferred hand, which is on the same (ipsilateral) side as the stored movement representations, would have only indirect access to these representations, via the corpus callosum. Decades later, researchers found that when learning a new skill the hand opposite the hemisphere that stores movement representations would also have an advantage over the hand that can get only indirect access to them.

Disorders of the brain that cause weakness, sensory loss, or shaking can impair a patient's ability to perform skilled movements. But Liepmann first described a different movement disorder, one characterized by spatial and temporal movement errors. He called this disorder ideomotor limb apraxia. Research nearly a century later confirmed that this disorder is caused by destruction of the movement representations or a disconnection of the representations from motor areas of the brain that control the limbs.

Brain imaging studies of right-handed patients with brain injuries and normal subjects provide evidence that movement representations, which store knowledge of the spatial and temporal patterns that are required to perform a skilled act, are stored in the inferior parietal lobe of the left hemisphere. Most right-handed patients who develop ideomotor apraxia have left-hemisphere injuries. Although the left hemisphere is important for speech and language, apraxia in right-handers does not always correspond with speech and language problems, and vice versa. Thus, these two brain systems are somewhat independent. There have been similar findings in left-handed patients who have apraxia from injury to their right hemisphere. There are, however, also rare reports of right-handed patients who developed both apraxia and speech problems after a stroke in their right hemisphere. These reports suggest that neither language laterality nor laterality of movement representations—nor even a combination of the two—can entirely account for my preference to throw with my right hand.

DEFTNESS-DEXTERITY

Billy Cox, the third baseman that the Dodgers got from Pittsburgh, was a great fielder because he had quick hands. Even after a well-hit ball took a bad hop, he could move his hands rapidly and accurately into the correct position, catch the ball, and throw the batter out at first. In addition, great pitchers throw a variety of pitches with similar arm motions. These different pitches rely on the spin of the ball, and the spins are made by alterations of the finger positions. The ability to perform precise, rapid, independent, but coordinated finger and hand movements is called deftness.

Tests of hand-finger deftness include rapid finger tapping; rapid rotation of a coin between the thumb, forefinger, and middle finger; and picking up pegs and placing them in holes. Studies of humans and monkeys suggest that these elemental motor skills depend on the integrity of what is called the corticospinal motor system. The nerve cells in this system reside in the motor cortex, which is at the back of the frontal lobes. These motor neurons have long axons, which are like wires that travel down through the brain and into the spinal cord. These neurons instruct the motor neurons in the spinal cord when to fire, and the firing of these spinal motor neurons makes specific muscles contract.

To learn whether structural asymmetries between the brain's hemispheres can help explain hand deftness and hand preference, my colleagues and I performed a study assessing structural hemispheric asymmetries of the motor cortex. We studied thirty subjects, fifteen who were right-handed and fifteen who were left-handed. Using magnetic resonance imaging (MRI), we measured the surface area of the hand and arm motor regions in these subjects' brains. We found that right-handed people had a larger motor cortex in the hand area of their left hemisphere than their right. In the left-handed people, however, we did not find a corresponding asymmetry—the motor cortex in the hand area of the right hemisphere was not larger. Although deftness asymmetries often are not as great in left- as right-handed people, this anomaly has not been explained. In any case, these results suggest that asymmetries of the motor cortex may be responsible for differences in hand deftness, and asymmetries of hand deftness might contribute to hand preference.

These asymmetries might play a critical role in the hand a person selects to perform activities such as writing or buttoning. Research has shown that throwing a ball requires movement knowledge and finger precision. But it remains unclear how asymmetries of deftness might influence whether a person bats left- or right-handed.

OTHER HEMISPHERIC ASYMMETRIES

When a right-handed batter stands at the plate, he must look to the left to see the pitcher. Research in 1990 showed that when seeing something on the right side, the brain of right-handed people primarily prepares the right hand for action, but seeing something on the left side causes the brain to prepare both hands for action. Because hitters hold the bat with both hands, standing to the left of home plate and watching the pitcher's delivery allows the right-handed batter to prepare both hands for action. We suspect that research would reveal a mirror version of these findings in left-handed people, but they have not been studied.

A study performed in our laboratory about five years later

suggests that whereas the left hemisphere has a bias to attend to stimuli that are close to the body (proximal bias), the right hemisphere has a bias to attend to stimuli that are far from the body (distal bias). Thus, when right-handed batters stand to the left of home plate and look leftward, their attention is focused far from the body (distally) on the pitcher. This allows them to see the pitcher's windup and delivery and prepare both hands for action.

POSTURES

When attempting to bat left-handed I was repeatedly told, "Make certain that your right hand is below your left." After putting my right hand around the lower portion of the bat and my left hand above my right I remember feeling terribly uncomfortable. This posture just did not feel correct. I also remember asking one of the coaches why people who bat right-handed like to keep the right hand above their left hand. He said, "This way the right hand is closer to where the action takes place." As indicated above, in most right-handed people this preferred hand is defter (more dexterous) than the left and can also better perform complex movements. Thus, keeping the right hand closer to the "business end" of the bat might allow better control.

The explanation did not entirely account for why right-handed people, when performing other sports, have different postures than left-handed people. For example, when I learned to box, the coach taught me to stand very similar to the way I stood when batting right-handed: sideways with my left foot forward. I was told to keep my right fist close to my chest and my left arm partially extended toward the opponent. I was also told that this posture would allow me to jab with my left hand and to save my right hand for the knockout punch. In addition, it would allow me to use my right arm to block my opponent's punches. This made sense. My right arm was stronger than my left, and the farther this right fist could travel before hitting my opponent, the greater the speed it could reach. In addition, my right arm—faster and able to carry out more precise movements than my left—should do a better job of blocking my opponent's punches.

When I went to a summer camp I was taught to shoot a bow and arrow, and later a rifle. I again was taught as a right-hander to take a stance similar to the one I used when batting and boxing: left foot forward, left arm extended, right arm flexed. When shooting a bow and arrow, a right-handed person might need the strength of his right arm to draw the bowstring, but when shooting a rifle it is the left hand that is closer to the business end. In addition, when using a shovel, rake, or hoe it is usually the left hand that is closer to the business end. These observations suggest that the coach's explanation about keeping my dominant hand closer to the business end does not account for why right-handed people keep their right hand above the left when holding the bat, nor does it entirely explain right-handed people's postures during other types of two-handed activities. The business end idea also does not explain why just holding the bat with my right hand below the left while my arms rotated over the left shoulder felt so uncomfortable and so unnatural.

Recently my colleagues and I proposed that there might be an alternative explanation for postures taken in all these sports. As mentioned above, whereas the right hemisphere appears to have a distal spatial attentional bias, the left has a proximal attentional bias. Action and postural biases are often parallel to attentional biases. When the right-handed hitter prepares to hit the ball (the ready position), his arms are rotated to the right side of the body, and in this ready position the right hand is closer to the body than the left hand is. In all the activities mentioned above, such as boxing and shooting, the right-handed person keeps the right arm closer to the body than they keep the left hand. Perhaps the left hemisphere has not only a proximal attentional bias but also a proximal motor-postural bias that allows it to better control the right hand when that hand is close to the body.

To assess this possibility, my colleagues and I had right-handed people hold pens in both their left and right hands, place the pen points on the left and right side of a page, and attempt to draw, with their eyes closed, horizontal lines that were parallel to their chest. We found that right-handed participants had a propensity for their right hand to move closer to their body than did the left hand. This observation provides support for the idea that the left hemisphere likes to keep the right hand close to the body. Thus, when right-handed people perform activities with both hands they have the propensity to keep their right hand closer to their bodies. This might explain why, when using implements such as a shovel, most right-handed people keep their left hand closer to the business end and their right hand closer to their body.

LEFT-HANDED BATTERS

Although we have mentioned some of the reasons why right-handed batters might hold the bat and stand as they do, we have not fully discussed the possible reasons why many of the greatest hitters who have played in the major leagues are left-handed.

The first explanation for the superiority of the left-handed batters is that left-handed people are not just the reverse of right-handed people. There are several questionnaires used to assess hand preference, such as the Edinburgh and the Waterloo Handedness questionnaires. When a large group of people are asked questions about their hand preference, the vast majority reveal that they prefer their right hand for tasks that require only one hand. A smaller group prefer the left hand. Although individuals in each group have differences in their consistency of preference, the people who overall prefer to use their right hand use it for almost everything they do with one hand. In contrast, the people who overall prefer to use their left hand also use their right hand for many activities that require the use of just one hand. These results suggest that people who overall prefer to use their left hand have the better ability to skillfully use either hand. When performing activities that require the skilled use of both hands, such as batting, having two hands that can make skillful movements provides an advantage. Thus, because left-handed people are in general more ambidextrous than right-handed people, the lefties might be more likely to be outstanding hitters.

There is an alternative, but not mutually exclusive, hypothesis that might explain the overall superiority of left-handed hitters: eye dominance. In addition to having excellent motor control, a great batter also has to have great vision. They have to be able to accurately perceive the speed of the ball and its trajectory, with what are called visuospatial skills. As mentioned above, in right-handed people the left hemisphere is dominant for mediating speech and language, but the right hemisphere is dominant for visuospatial functions. Studies of patients with lesions of the left or right hemisphere have revealed that this same asymmetry—left/verbal, right/visuospatial—also occurs in the majority of left-handed people. Moreover, while the left hemisphere primarily attends to the space immediately around us, the right hemisphere has a propensity to attend to the space farther away from our body. The hitter watches the pitcher with both eyes, but most people have a dominant eye. For a visual task such as hitting a baseball, the batter is more likely to use the visual information from this dominant eye than from the non-dominant eye.

Hand and eye dominance do not always correlate, but left-handed people are more likely to be left-eye dominant than are right-handed people. Although each eye projects to both the left and right hemispheres, each eye has stronger projections to the opposite hemisphere. My colleagues and I demonstrated that when using the right eye, subjects' attention is biased toward the space that is nearest to their body, but when using their left eye, their attention is biased to the space farther away from their body. Left-eye dominance might allow greater visual input into the right hemisphere, which directs attention to far space—the sixty feet, six inches between home plate and the pitcher's mound, for example. These hemispheric asymmetries might help left-handed hitters, who are more likely to be left-eye dominant, better attend to the pitcher and the early trajectory of the ball as well as make superior visuospatial computations. These attentional and visuospatial advantages might allow the left-handed batter to more successfully compute the trajectory of the pitched ball.

THROWING AND CATCHING

When I was learning to catch with my baseball glove, my dad and brother told me that I had to wear the glove on my left hand, because then I could throw the ball with my right hand. This explanation seemed reasonable until I started writing this chapter and thought to myself, "Does it really require more skill to throw than catch, or do right-handed ballplayers catch with the left hand and throw with the right because these two hands, which are primarily controlled by different hemispheres, have different types of skills?"

Clearly, throwing a ball requires greater finger deftness than catching a ball with a baseball glove. As mentioned, in almost all right-handed people the right hand and fingers are defter than the left. When catching a ball, one of the most important functions is aligning the glove so that the pocket of the glove is aligned with the ball when the ball enters the fielder's immediate space. This type of alignment would appear to be more heavily dependent on visuospatial skills. The right hemisphere, which primarily controls the left hand and arm, appears to be dominant in mediating visuospatial skills; thus, there might be a slight advantage for right-handed people to catch balls with their gloved left hand.

In any case, I have given up trying to hit or throw left-handed, but I have not given up trying to learn more about handedness. I am planning to perform additional studies to test some of the hypotheses discussed in this chapter, but for the moment these plans are in the realm of the fan's dejected sigh: "Wait 'til next year."

-7-

IT ISN'T WHETHER YOU WIN
OR LOSE, IT'S WHETHER YOU WIN

Agony and Ecstasy in the Brain

KELLI WHITLOCK BURTON AND
HILLARY R. RODMAN, PH.D.

In October 2003, Cubs fans had reason to believe their long-standing loyalty would finally be rewarded. After defeating the Atlanta Braves on October 5 to win a postseason series for the first time since 1908, the Cubs would play the Florida Marlins for the National League title and a chance to compete in their first World Series in nearly sixty years.

Cubs faithful came early to Wrigley Field on October 7 for the first game against the Marlins, only to see their team lose in extra innings. The Cubs bounced back, however, winning the next three games—including an extra-inning win in Miami in game 3 on October 10. By game 5, the Cubs were just one win away from capturing the National League pennant. But the Marlins won that game 4–0.

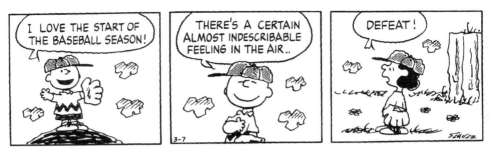

Peanuts: © United Feature Syndicate, Inc.

Still, the Cubs returned home with two more chances to advance to the Fall Classic. Nearly 40,000 Cubs fans cheered as their team emerged from the home dugout to begin game 6. Thousands more followed the game on television, radio, and the Internet.

In the top of the eighth inning with one out, the Cubs led the Marlins 3–0 and were just five outs away from a return to the World Series. Marlins second baseman Luis Castillo hit a foul ball toward the left field seats. As if in a bad dream, fans watched helplessly as Cubs outfielder Moises Alou's attempt to catch the ball was foiled by an eager fan. Castillo went on to draw a walk, setting off an eight-run scoring frenzy that led to a Marlins victory. The Cubs could not turn the tide and lost game 7. It was the Marlins, not the Northsiders, who went on to face the New York Yankees in the 2003 World Series— and win.

The road from ecstasy to agony took less than two weeks to travel, with many smaller peaks and valleys en route. It's a path familiar to legions of Cubs fans and to followers of other baseball teams as well, albeit with varying ratios of despair to delight. The outward display of emotion is easy to document. But what of the cascade of mechanisms in the brain activated by emotions linked to anticipation and disappointment?

In recent years, scientists have been aided by new technologies that are helping to answer some old questions about how the brain processes negative and positive experiences of the type familiar—sometimes all *too* familiar—to the baseball fan. They are gaining insight into emotion, memory, social behavior, prognostication of future events, and the processes that psychologists refer to as reward and punishment. Studies on these topics, which involve research on depression, sadness, grief, and euphoria, provide data about changes in brain activity under a variety of conditions and emotional states. Some of these conditions may cause only temporary alterations in function in regions of the brain involved in emotion and, to some degree, certain areas that deal with physical pain. Others, such as drug addiction, can result in long-term changes in both neural sensitivity and structure. Is it possible, then, that the long-suffering fan of a team prone to snatching defeat from the jaws of victory likewise has subtle and long-lasting changes in his or her brain reward circuitry, comparable to a kind of addiction?

LIFE, LOSS, AND BASEBALL

In her 1969 book, *On Death and Dying,* psychiatrist Elisabeth Kübler-Ross described five stages of grief: denial, anger, bargaining, depression, and acceptance. While originally applied only to the loss of a loved one, psychologists today often apply Kübler-Ross's stages to a variety of tragic experiences in an individual's life, ranging from the loss of a job to the breakup of a marriage. Given the importance that society bestows on sports and athletic performance, it seems appropriate to apply these stages to a beleaguered fan. When the Cubs lost after having a 3–1 series lead against the Marlins in 2003, Cubs fans were stunned; this couldn't be happening. Denial gave way quickly to anger, and the fans' target was the fan who had made a play on the foul ball in game 6, a man named Steve Bartman. The attacks began as Bartman, shielding himself from debris and obscenities hurled by fans who believed he was to blame for the team's downfall, was led out of Wrigley Field under protective guard. Bartman's name, address, phone number, and place of employment were published the following day by the *Chicago Sun-Times,* and hate mail and death threats ensued. Even Illinois governor Rod Blagojevich vented his frustration, suggesting that Bartman consider joining a witness protection program.

Emotions have immediate, visceral components—such as the heart rate and adrenaline surge baseball fans might experience while watching their team's shot at a World Series slip away. But emotions also have a more thought-based or cognitive component that comes into play—a fan's reflection on the ethics of the governor's suggestion, for example. In general, emotion can be thought of as a collaboration between a set of structures deep in the brain called the limbic system and the most forward part of the outer covering of the brain in the frontal lobes, the prefrontal cortex. Relative to other animals, humans have a disproportionately large prefrontal cortex, which helps to explain our ability to plan, to reason, and to experience subtle variations of feeling. In healthy individuals, the limbic system and specific parts of the prefrontal cortex interact with brain regions that control action. In doing so, they help put a specific pleasant or unpleasant "stamp" on existing memories, which helps tie ongoing events to existing memories.

For Cubs fans, memories of the 2003 National League Championship Series carry a particularly unpleasant stamp. The days leading up to the final games held such hope, such promise, that a post-series crash seemed almost inevitable. As a result, some fans may have been lethargic, sad, or hopeless. More extreme reactions might even have included a loss of appetite, sleep disturbances, and a lack of interest in formerly desirable activities. Many of these symptoms have been documented and studied at length in patients with clinical depression. While most grieving sports fans do not suffer from depression, it is worthwhile to examine research in the field to get a better sense of what might be happening in the brains of distressed fans.

With the advent of technology such as functional magnetic resonance imaging, researchers have been able to identify which regions in the brain are associated with a variety of functions, including the experience of emotion. Within the human prefrontal cortex, scientists have distinguished several subareas: a lateral prefrontal region on the side of the brain; an orbitofrontal region that nestles around the eye sockets; and a ventromedial region, which lies on the bottom and midline surfaces of the hemisphere. Whereas the lateral prefrontal cortex seems to play a role in choosing courses of action, the orbitofrontal and ventromedial regions are implicated more directly in emotion. In depressed patients, the ventromedial prefrontal cortex (and other prefrontal regions to a lesser extent) shows a decrease in activity. It has even been reported that the ventromedial cortex is smaller in patients with a hereditary form of depression.

In contrast to the decreased activity seen in the prefrontal cortex, a limbic structure called the amygdala, deep within the temporal lobe, shows abnormally high activity in depressed patients. The amygdala appears to play an especially important role in detecting negative stimuli and producing negative states such as fear (though it is increasingly seen as involved in pleasant emotions as well). Thus, hyperactivity in this structure might be responsible for the anxiety and misperception of stimuli as threatening that depressed patients often show.

In addition to the prefrontal cortex and the amygdala, there is a strip of more primitive cortex located along the edge of the cerebral hemisphere where the two hemispheres meet, at the midline above the brain stem. Called the cingulate cortex, this region is also heavily implicated in emotion, as well as in other functions. Overall, the cingulate cortex has been reported to be less active in depressed patients, but its front-most part, like the amygdala, shows increased activity in some studies. Finally, depressed patients show decreased activity in a structure called the ventral striatum, part of the brain's reward circuit, and changes in a deeply buried region of the cortex called the insula, a region involved in all types of subjectively unpleasant experiences.

It is tempting to speculate that the disappointed baseball fan experiences a set of brain changes analogous to those described above for people with depression. However, few of even the most die-hard fans experience behavioral and psychological changes severe enough to warrant a formal diagnosis of major depression. Accordingly, studies of the experience of negative emotions of a more time-limited or less overwhelming nature may provide additional insight into the brain of the long-suffering fan who nevertheless continues to function well in other spheres of life. Studies of induced sadness offer a good model.

Sadness has been of interest to psychologists both as an emotional state and as a forerunner of more severe clinical conditions. Most studies attempt to cultivate a sad mood in participants by asking them to recall a sad memory, by showing them movies with sad themes, or by presenting pictures of human faces with unhappy expressions. These types of conditions might be considered comparable to the recent experience of a single lost game or a more distant memory of an especially devastating one. On the other hand, studies of grief following separation from a loved one might be more relevant to the emotions surrounding the end of a once-promising season.

While there are numerous studies of induced sadness, there have only been a few to date investigating grief. A 2004 study in Germany by researcher Arif Najib and colleagues examined brain activity in women grieving the breakup of a romantic relationship. Such an experience—with its components of sudden loss and the need to renounce imaginings of a specific rosy future—holds some similarities to that of a fan coping with the abrupt end of his team's season with a loss in the playoffs. Subjects in this study showed alterations in most of the brain regions implicated in real physical pain, some of which are also implicated in clinical depression. Subjects who reported higher levels of grief showed greater changes in almost all of these regions, suggesting that the subjective impact of the relevant events had direct implications for brain function.

Researchers also have studied what are called social defeat and social stress, which provide fascinating insights into how life events can lead to the development of hopelessness and depression. Although it is the players who experience social defeat directly, there is ample reason to believe that fans' emotional investment in and identification with their teams cause changes in their nervous and hormonal systems.

In laboratory rats and other rodents, social defeat is typically studied by introducing one male animal (the intruder) briefly into the home cage of another, aggressive male (the resident). The resident then attacks and "defeats" the intruder, who then seems changed: interest in running on a wheel and in going exploring decreases, while "anxiety" in situations where it feels unprotected (such as on an elevated runway with open edges) increases. The consequences in these animals' brains have been studied at many levels, and in some cases they are similar to changes revealed by brain imaging in humans. For example, defeat in a circumstance such as the intruder-resident attack above is followed by the expression of a protein in brain areas that can be activated by physically painful stimuli or other types of stress.

Evidently, social defeat is highly effective in producing a state analogous to psychological pain in animals. Interestingly, both the behavioral and the brain effects of social defeat are greatest when defeated animals are housed individually, rather than with compatible cagemates. Indeed, animals with companionship may not experience these effects at all. Perhaps, like the disappointed baseball fan seeking commiseration after a bad loss, subsequent social support is crucial to the defeated rat in returning to a normal "state of mind."

Social defeat also has been studied in the context of long-term repercussions of negative experiences, especially when such experiences are repeated. Social defeat sets in motion a number of brain processes that lead to increased sensitivity to subsequent stressful experiences. Different brain areas that change after a single defeat show varying patterns after repeated defeat: some (especially in the brain stem) continue to be activated at a high rate with each new defeat, whereas others seem to adapt. Thus, different structures play different roles in the response to defeat. In addition, at least one structure—the hippocampus—actually changes physically after repeated defeat experiences. The hippocampus is well known to be crucial for the formation of memories of specific experiences, and its nerve cells show significant plasticity—the ability to change both structure and function—as animals learn. In addition, the hippocampus is one of a few structures that make new nerve cells in adulthood, a phenomenon known as neurogenesis. In rats, both repeated defeat (defeats on alternate days for several weeks) and a "double defeat" on successive days cause striking changes to the parts of cells in the hippocampus that receive incoming information from other regions of the brain. Moreover, both acute and persistent defeat decrease neurogenesis, and persistent defeat causes long-lasting changes in the ability of the same nerve cells to respond electrically to stimuli. Research has also begun to identify the chemical bases of long-lasting brain changes after social defeat, with the neurotransmitter serotonin—also heavily implicated in clinical depression—among the substances most clearly involved.

THEY DID IT! EUPHORIA IN THE BRAIN

In the fall of 2004, the Boston Red Sox made the biggest comeback in baseball history by snatching the American League Championship from the New York Yankees, who had won the first three games of the series and were just three outs away from sweeping their archenemy. The Sox won four straight games to capture the league pennant and then went on to win four more to sweep the St. Louis Cardinals in the World Series.

Some three million fans—known as the Red Sox Nation—took to the streets of Boston on October 30 for a parade to celebrate the city's first World Series victory in eighty-six years. Fans flew in from overseas just to catch a glimpse of the Red Sox players as they rode past in amphibious vehicles. Weddings were postponed, bar mitzvahs rescheduled, school field trips missed. News reports described the event as "euphoric," a long-awaited triumph for Red Sox fans, who had suffered many heartbreaking late-season and postseason losses.

The sensation of euphoria seems to originate in the pit of the stomach, the good vibes emanating from the gut and traveling to every nerve in the body, resulting in wide smiles, wildly clapping hands, and boisterous cheers. However, the set of events that includes that giddiness also involves the brain's "reward circuit." Vertebrate brains are equipped with a built-in mechanism for feeling a sense of pleasure from activities that are intrinsically useful, such as eating food or mating. In human beings, the same system is also activated by more esoteric and diverse activities such as satisfying curiosity, taking certain types of drugs, engaging in social contact, and, presumably, more cerebral pursuits such as viewing a fine painting, winning a game of chess, or seeing one's favorite team put an end to an eighty-six-year dry spell with a World Series victory.

First identified by James Olds and Peter Milner in the 1950s, the reward circuit begins in a region of the midbrain called the ventral tegmental area. In their experiments, Olds and Milner discovered that rats would work diligently to press a lever that would send tiny jolts of electricity into the parts of the brain mentioned above, as if activating the nerve cells in those structures somehow made the rats feel good. Nowadays, the concept of reward is especially prevalent in research related to drug addiction. For example, ingestion of stimulant drugs such as cocaine, amphetamine, or Ecstasy has been shown in rats to release dopamine into the brain, presumably producing the same brain state that Olds and Milner saw in their rats. Moreover, taking such drugs over long periods of time produces long-term changes in the sensitivity of the reward system, and current work focuses on trying to understand exactly how such changes take place.

As any fan knows, following the sport of choice can produce a number of different good feelings. One component is undoubtedly the rich and acute enjoyment of a major positive turn of events, such as an important win over a rival team or an incredible string of victories in September and October. Another component, heightened by background knowledge, is the anticipation of such positive outcomes. In the case of baseball, the immense role played by statistics and history reflects the overall importance of this second type of enjoyment—made all the more relevant nowadays by the availability of unlimited baseball information and data on the Internet. Similar distinctions can be made, however, for other types of rewarding experiences. In fact, neuroscientists who study reward often draw a distinction between the hedonic impact, or pleasure of actually having the reward, and the anticipation of getting it, which points to how well the reward serves as an incentive to motivate behavior. To some extent, these aspects of reward can be dissociated within the brain as well.

In seeking to understand the components of enjoyment, Johns Hopkins University researchers Peter Holland and Michela Gallagher emphasize the interaction between two specific components of the human reward system, the orbitofrontal cortex (OFC) and the amygdala. Within the OFC, separate regions seem to play differing roles in reward, with more lateral parts of the OFC actually more involved in evaluating negative or punishing events, according to Morten Kringelbach at the University of Oxford in the United Kingdom. Within the more medial, reward-related component of the orbitofrontal cortex, several additional distinctions can be drawn. The part of the medial OFC that lies farther back tends to become active when subjects are given simple rewards such as food, whereas the portions of the medial OFC nearer the front are stimulated when the rewards are more abstract or complex ones, such as money, praise, or music. In other words, one area of the OFC is activated in the brain of a fan savoring a Fenway Frank, but a different area switches on when the fan looks up to see his team complete a rare triple play.

What about expectation itself, one of the crucial subjective components of enjoyment? To study this aspect, neuroscientist Hans Breiter and colleagues at Harvard University Medical School gave participants $50 and taught them to play a game of chance in which they might make more money, lose all the money, or break even. Using functional magnetic resonance imaging, the researchers showed that the prospect of gaining or losing money activates both a portion of the OFC and a region near the amygdala. Followers of an underdog team know well the added sweetness, albeit rare, of an unexpected win (a concept neatly encapsulated in the sports betting conceit of "against the spread"). Human brain imaging studies indicate that activation of the OFC by rewards is consistently greater when cues in the experimental situation cause us to hope for the reward without being able to predict it. Finally, Michael Cohen and colleagues at the University of California, Davis, have shown that individual differences in both extraversion and hereditary brain chemistry predict differences in the magnitude of the brain's response to rewards— but not anticipation of them. Specifically, more outgoing individuals were likely to show stronger brain responses to the actual delivery of a reward. A similar relationship was found between having a particular genetic marker related to the neurotransmitter dopamine. This marker is associated with addictive disorders and strong reward responses. Thus, being especially susceptible to the actual experience of pleasure may depend at least in part on personality variables and heredity. It is tempting to speculate that teams that always seem to do well might draw fans of specific types, but no such research has been conducted.

But what of a team that goes from worst to the World Series during the same season, such as the 2007 Colorado Rockies and 1992 Atlanta Braves? Both teams were in last place early on and remained near the bottom for much of the summer. But then something unexpected happened: They started to win. Unlike supporters of other teams that played well for the entire season, fans of the Rockies and Braves were thrust into a state of growing euphoria as their teams battled back. In a last-to-first situation, it is worth asking if the nervous system registers certain types of special or peak experiences differently than more routinely rewarding ones. In fact, scientists have been interested in just this question.

Probably the most common model of euphoria in humans involves the assessment of brain function during drug ingestion by addicted individuals—cocaine addicts experiencing a cocaine rush, for example. Different patterns of activation are produced during cocaine craving (before taking the drug) and cocaine euphoria (after the drug is ingested). In a study led by Harvard's Hans Breiter, an addict who took cocaine showed increased activity in a large subset of areas belonging to the networks for emotion and reward. A 2001 study that did not involve drugs investigated brain activity in people listening to music (of their own selection) so highly pleasurable that they consistently reported the experience as provoking physical "chills" or "shivers down the spine." The research, led by Anne Blood and Robert Zatorre at McGill University in Montreal, Canada, employed an older type of functional imaging called positron emission tomography to compare each subject's brain activity during the "chills" experience with that obtained when the subject heard music selected by others. Overall, the data suggest that intensely pleasurable experiences strongly activate neural circuits implicated in reward and emotion but do not establish a special "signature" to distinguish them from other types of pleasurable experiences.

A different way of conceptualizing the involvement of a baseball fan with his or her team is to draw on parallels between fanmanship and the practice of religious faith. (For a different angle on religion, see Chapter 4.) In an eloquent essay on this topic, University of Arkansas philosophy professor Thomas Senor argues that Cubs fans in particular have much to teach us about the nature of faith and commitment. Similarly to devoted practitioners of many religions, fans suspend disbelief in the face of contradictory evidence, engage in ritualistic practices, struggle with their faith, hold on to eternal hope, and, on occasion, experience sublime satisfaction associated with these activities. Thus, it may also be worthwhile to examine the small but growing body of research investigating neural correlates of religious experience. Historically, views of the brain and religion implicated the temporal lobes, in part because of the similarity between hallucinations induced by temporal lobe seizures and descriptions of religious visions. To test this idea, in 2003 the well-known evolutionary biologist Richard Dawkins agreed to have his temporal lobes stimulated using a technique called transcranial magnetic stimulation, in the hope of eliciting a mystical experience. None, however, was produced. Today, interest in the neural correlates of religion has expanded beyond the temporal lobe, and the most compelling data may, in fact, implicate other regions of the brain.

In one study led by University of Hawaii psychology professor Nina P. Azari, self-identified religious subjects reciting psalms activated primarily the lateral prefrontal cortex and portions of both the medial frontal lobe and the medial portion of the parietal lobe, regions associated with sustaining reflective thought. It was notable in Azari's study that limbic areas most associated with emotion were not activated, suggesting that at least for the religious activity studied, the mental or cognitive component, rather than the emotional one, may be crucial. In later work, however, Azari and colleagues showed that religious experience was expressed in both a frontal network and in a subset of the cortical areas important for reward, action preparation, and emotion-related language processing. (Ritual recitation of "Take Me Out to the Ball Game" has yet to be studied.)

Scientists have also examined the neurochemistry of religious experience. The neurotransmitter serotonin has been of special interest because drugs such as LSD and mescaline, which produce hallucinations, alter brain serotonin function. In imaging research by a team of Swedish researchers led by Jörgen Borg, subjects who scored high on tests of self-transcendence (a personality trait that takes into account both religious behavior and attitudes) had low scores on a measure of brain serotonin activity. These authors suggest that because serotonin has a role in shutting down arousal and sensory stimulation, low serotonin activity might better allow for appreciation of sensory stimuli not otherwise experienced. Although religious inclination and the ability to appreciate the subtle beauties of baseball may or may not correlate, data on brain mechanisms of religious experience suggest a more purely reflective component that might well be crucial in appreciating the complexities of history and circumstance that accompany each pitch in a professional baseball game.

IN HIS CLEATS: VICARIOUS EMOTIONS

A primary component of fanmanship is the tendency to identify, consciously or not, with the individuals who play the game. Many Red Sox fans still feel a residual anger at the hapless Bill Buckner, the Red Sox first baseman who let a ground ball roll through his legs in game 6 of the 1986 World Series, allowing the Mets to score the winning run. So intense is Boston's displeasure with Buckner that the Leonard P. Zakim Bunker Hill Bridge, a cable-suspended bridge that takes eight lanes of traffic through the center of an inverted Y–shaped structure across the Charles River in Boston, has been nicknamed the "Buckner Bridge." The 2004 World Series victory (and another in 2007) went a long way toward healing these old wounds, but most Sox fans shared in the dismay that Buckner undoubtedly experienced as he turned to see the ball behind him—a feeling most sports fans can relate to. In short, we empathize, and we experience covertly the emotional states that our players do.

Increasingly, scientists are gaining an appreciation for the effectiveness with which covert experience activates the brain of the observer to simulate the mental state of the individuals observed. For example, we now know that there are special neurons in a monkey's brain that fire not only when it performs a specific action (such as reaching out), but also when it simply sits still and watches another monkey perform the same task. Called mirror neurons, they are found primarily in the parts of the cortex that control or plan movements, such as the premotor cortex. This holds true for humans, according to imaging studies. Other human imaging research suggests that our brains can also simulate inferred emotional states. For example, French scientist Bruno Wicker and colleagues studied brain activity as humans smelled unpleasant or neutral substances. They then tracked changes in the brain when subjects observed another person looking into a cup, then grimacing in disgust. Even though subjects smelled nothing in the second experiment, a region in the front part of the insula reacted similarly under both conditions, perhaps providing the neural basis of the imagined experience.

Moving directly into the realm of sports fanmanship, there is evidence that sports fans react physically to game outcomes in much the same way as the players. Winning or losing a contest or battle causes hormonal changes, notably shifts in the production of testosterone. For example, when male rats defend their territory against invading rats, the defeated animals show predictable and significant declines in circulating testosterone levels immediately after the contest. Winning individuals or team members, on the other hand, show increases. In a 1998 study, University of Utah scientist Paul Bernhardt and colleagues found that male sports fans who witnessed their teams win or lose experienced changes in testosterone levels similar to those of the players. Bernhardt's subjects were soccer and basketball fans, but it is likely that results in baseball fans would be similar. These studies suggest that the vicarious experiences of the sports fan—whether suffering through a defeat or celebrating a win—have a strong basis in the endocrine system as well as the brain. In short, empathy is not only a psychological concept, but also a physical phenomenon.

HOPE SPRINGS ETERNAL

The ecstasy and despair of the committed baseball fan are real, deep emotions that add richness and complexity to life. However, only rarely do these feelings lead to a pattern of behavior and emotion that negatively impact an individual's ability to cope with daily life. Indeed, fanmanship allows us to partake of events with high emotional salience but limited finality. After all, one of the finest characteristics of baseball is the opportunity for constant renewal. One day's game is wiped out in the promise of the next; one season is always followed by another; a retiring player is replaced by a youngster who might—just might—turn out to be the rookie phenom not seen in ages. Highs and lows are a desirable part of life to most of us; in fact, manic-depressive patients sometimes forgo their medications because the emotional dulling is not worth the behavioral balance the treatment brings. In following teams that provide a lifetime of near successes, Cubs fans and others have perhaps perfected the art of experiencing highs and lows while keeping high expectation and hope for the savor of the richest reward. What, then, will happen when the Northsiders finally win it all? A newspaper article published after the Red Sox captured the 2004 World Series told of an elderly Sox fan who, just after the glorious day for which he had waited a lifetime, stated that he could now die a man at peace. Undoubtedly, upon the Cubs ascension, some fans—no matter their age—will feel the same way. The majority, undoubtedly, will stick with their (former) "Lovable Losers." But it might not be surprising to hear from at least a few:

"Perhaps it's time to root for the Royals."

REFERENCES

CHAPTER 1

Abrams, D., and M. A. Hogg. (1988). Comments on the motivational status of self-esteem in social identity and intergroup discrimination. *European Journal of Social Psychology* 18: 317–334.

Gallese, V. (2007). Embodied simulation: From mirror neuron systems to interpersonal relations. In *Empathy and fairness,* 3–12. Novartis Foundation Symposium 278. Chichester, UK: John Wiley & Sons.

Green, C. D. (2003). Psychology strikes out: Coleman R. Griffith and the Chicago Cubs. *History of Psychology* 6(3): 267–283.

Insel, T. R. (2003). Is social attachment an addictive disorder? *Physiology and Behavior* 79(3): 351–357.

Kosfeld, M., M. Heinrichs, P. J. Zak, U. Fischbacher, and E. Fehr. (2005). Oxytocin increases trust in humans. *Nature* 435(7042): 673–676.

Kruglanski, A. W., and E. T. Higgins, eds. (2007). *Social psychology: Handbook of basic principles.* 2d ed. New York: Guilford Press.

Kunda, Z. (1987). Motivated inference: Self-serving generation and evaluation of causal theories. *Journal of Personality and Social Psychology* 53(4): 636–647.

Levine, J. M., and R. L. Moreland. (1994). Group socialization: Theory and research. In *European review of social psychology,* vol. 5, ed. W. Stroebe and M. Hewstone, 305–336. Chichester, UK: John Wiley & Sons.

Lieberman, M. D. (2007). Social cognitive neuroscience: A review of core processes. *Annual Review of Psychology* 58: 259–289.

Mischel, W., Y. Shoda, and M. L. Rodriguez. (1989). Delay of gratification in children. *Science* 244: 933–938.

Moll, J., R. Zahn, R. de Oliveira-Souza, F. Krueger, and J. Grafman. (2005). Opinion: The neural basis of human moral cognition. *Nature Reviews Neuroscience* 6(10): 799–809.

Murray, S. L., and J. G. Holmes. (1993). Seeing virtues in faults: Negativity and the transformation of interpersonal narratives in close relationships. *Journal of Personality and Social Psychology* 65(4): 707–722.

Nemeth, C. J. (1986). Differential contributions of majority and minority influence. *Psychological Review* 93(1): 23–32.

Reid, A., and K. Deaux. (1997). Relationship between social and personal identities: Segregation or integration? *Journal of Personality and Social Psychology* 71: 1084–1091.

Risberg, J., and J. Grafman, eds. (2006). *The frontal lobes: Development, function and pathology.* Cambridge: Cambridge University Press.

CHAPTER 2

Cross, E. S., A. F. de C. Hamilton, and S. T. Grafton. (2006). Building a motor simulation de novo: Observation of dance by dancers. *NeuroImage* 31(3): 1257–1267.

Ericsson, K. A., R. T. Krampe, and S. Heizmann. (1993). Can we create gifted people? In *The origins and development of high ability*, 222–231; discussion 232–249. Ciba Foundation Symposia 178. Chichester, UK: John Wiley & Sons.

Ericsson, K. A., and A. C. Lehmann. (1996). Expert and exceptional performance: Evidence of maximal adaptation to task constraints. *Annual Review of Psychology* 47: 273–305.

Gaser, C., and G. Schlaug. (2003). Brain structures differ between musicians and non-musicians. *Journal of Neuroscience* 23(27): 9240–9245.

Hamilton, A. F. de C., and S. T. Grafton. (2006). Goal representation in human anterior intraparietal sulcus. *Journal of Neuroscience* 26(4): 1133–1137.

Jäncke, L., N. J. Shah, and M. Peters. (2000). Cortical activations in primary and secondary motor areas for complex bimanual movements in professional pianists. *Cognitive Brain Research* 10(1–2): 177–183.

Koeneke, S., K. Lutz, T. Wüstenberg, and L. Jäncke. (2004). Long-term training affects cerebellar processing in skilled keyboard players. *NeuroReport* 15(8): 1279–1282.

McIntosh, A. R. (1999). Mapping cognition to the brain through neural interactions. *Memory* 7(5–6): 523–548.

Pascual-Leone, A. (2001). The brain that plays music and is changed by it. *Annals of the New York Academy of Science* 930: 315–329.

CHAPTER 3

Adair, R. K. (2002). *The physics of baseball.* 3d ed. New York: HarperCollins.

Albert, J., and J. Bennett. (2003). *Curve ball: Baseball, statistics, and the role of chance in the game.* Rev. ed. New York: Springer-Verlag.

Amassian, V. E., R. Q. Cracco, P. J. Maccabee, J. B. Cracco, A. P. Rudell, and L. Eberle. (1989). Suppression of visual perception by magnetic coil stimulation of human occipital cortex. *Electroencephalography and Clinical Neurophysiology* 74: 458–462.

Bartlett, R. (2000). Principles of throwing. In *Biomechanics in sport: Performance enhancement and injury prevention,* ed. V. M. Zatsiorsky, 365–380. The Encyclopaedia of Sports Medicine, 9. Malden, MA: Blackwell Science.

Beilock, S. L., and T. H. Carr. (2005). When high-powered people fail: Working memory and "choking under pressure" in math. *Psychological Science* 16(2): 101–105.

Binkofski, F., G. Buccino, S. Posse, R. J. Seitz, G. Rizzolatti, and H. J. Freund. (1999). A fronto-parietal circuit for object manipulation in man: Evidence from an fMRI-study. *European Journal of Neuroscience* 11: 3276–3286.

Churchland, M. M., A. Afshar, and K. V. Shenoy. (2006). A central source of movement variability. *Neuron* 52: 1085–1096.

Davidson, R. J., and W. Irwin. (1999). The functional neuroanatomy of emotion and affective style. *Trends in Cognitive Science* 3: 11–21.

Decety, J., M. Jeannerod, M. Germain, and J. Pastene. (1991). Vegetative response during imagined movement is proportional to mental effort. *Behavioural Brain Research* 42(1): 1–5.

Ding, S. L., R. J. Morecraft, and G. W. Van Hoesen. (2003). Topography, cytoarchitecture, and cellular phenotypes of cortical areas that form the cingulo-parahippocampal isthmus and adjoining retrocalcarine areas in the monkey. *Journal of Comparative Neurology* 456(2): 184–201.

Fairweather, M. (2003). Skill learning principles: Implications for coaching practice. In *The coaching process: Principles and practice for sport,* ed. N. Cross and J. Lyle, 113–129. Boston: Butterworth-Heinemann.

Fitts, P. M., and M. I. Posner. (1973). *Human performance.* London: Prentice/Hall International.

Gabbard, C. P. (2004). *Lifelong motor development.* 4th ed. New York: Benjamin Cummings.

Gibson, A. P., and R. D. Adams. (1989). Batting stroke timing with a bowler and a bowling machine: A case study. *Australian Journal of Science and Medicine in Sport* 21(2): 3–6.

Hatfield, B. D., and C. H. Hillman. (2001). The psychophysiology of sport: A mechanistic understanding of the psychology of superior performance. In *Handbook of sport psychology,* 2d ed., ed. R. N. Singer, H. A. Hausenblas, and C. M. Janelle, 362–386. New York: John Wiley & Sons.

Hick, W. E. (1952). On the rate of gain of information. *Quarterly Journal of Experimental Psychology* 4: 11–26.

James, B. (2001). *The new Bill James historical baseball abstract.* New York: Free Press.

Jeannerod, M., M. A. Arbib, G. Rizzolatti, and H. Sakata. (1995). Grasping objects: The cortical mechanisms of visuomotor transformation. *Trends in Neurosciences* 18(7): 314–320.

LeDoux, J. E. (2000). Emotion circuits in the brain. *Annual Review of Neuroscience* 23: 155–184.

Linder, D. E., R. Lutz, D. Crews, and M. Lochbaum. (1999). Who chokes and when? Situational and dispositional factors in failure under pressure. In *Science and Golf III: Proceedings of the World Scientific Congress of Golf,* ed. M. R. Farrally and A. J. Cochran, 207–212. Champaign, IL: Human Kinetics.

Magill, R. A. (1998). *Motor learning: Concepts and applications.* 5th ed. Boston: McGraw-Hill.

Mesulam, M. M., A. C. Nobre, Y. H. Kim, T. B. Parrish, and D. R. Gitelman. (2001). Heterogeneity of cingulate contributions to spatial attention. *NeuroImage* 13(6): 1065–1072.

Milton, J. G., S. L. Small, and A. Solodkin, editors. (2004a). Neurophysiology of skilled performance. *Journal of Clinical Neurophysiology* 21(3): 133–227.

———. (2004b). On the road to automatic: Dynamic aspects in the development of expertise. *Journal of Clinical Neurophysiology* 21(3): 134–143.

Milton, J., A. Solodkin, P. Hluštík, and S. L. Small. (2007). The mind of expert motor performance is cool and focused. *NeuroImage* 35: 804–813.

Müller, S., B. Abernethy, and D. Farrow. (2006). How do world-class cricket batsmen anticipate a bowler's intention? *Quarterly Journal of Experimental Psychology* 59(12): 2162–2186.

Mundel, T., J. G. Milton, A. Dimitrov, H. W. Wilson, C. Pelizzari, S. Uftring, I. Torres, R. K. Erikson, J. P. Spire, and V. L. Towle. (2003). Transient inability to distinguish between faces: Electrophysiologic studies. *Journal of Clinical Neurophysiology* 20(2): 102–110.

Oishi, K., T. Kasai, and T. Maeshima. (2000). Autonomic response specificity during motor imagery. *Journal of Physiological Anthropology and Applied Human Science* 19: 255–261.

Raichle, M. E., A. M. MacLeod, A. Z. Snyder, W. J. Powers, D. A. Gusnard, and G. L. Shulman. (2001). A default mode of brain function. *Proceedings of the National Academy of Sciences USA* 98(2): 676–682.

Rizzolatti, G., and L. Craighero. (2004). The mirror-neuron system. *Annual Review of Neuroscience* 27: 169–192.

Savelsbergh, G. J., A. M. Williams, J. Van der Kamp, and P. Ward. (2002). Visual search, anticipation and expertise in soccer goalkeepers. *Journal of Sports Sciences* 20(3): 279–287.

Schell, M. J. (2005). *Baseball's all-time best sluggers: Adjusted batting performance from strikeouts to home runs.* Princeton, NJ: Princeton University Press.

Schultz, R., D. Musa, J. Staszewski, and R. S. Seigler. (1994). The relationship between age and major league baseball performance: Implications for development. *Psychology and Aging* 9(2): 274–286.

Umiltà, M. A., E. Kohler, V. Gallese, L. Fogassi, L. Fadiga, C. Keysers, and G. Rizzolatti. (2001). I know what you are doing: A neurophysiological study. *Neuron* 31(1): 155–165.

CHAPTER 4

Boyer, P. (2002). *Religion explained: The evolutionary origins of religious thought.* New York: Basic Books.

Brugger, P. (2001). From haunted brain to haunted science: A cognitive neuroscience view of paranormal and pseudoscientific thought. In *Hauntings and poltergeists: Multidisciplinary perspectives,* ed. J. Houran and R. Lange, 195–213. Jefferson, NC: McFarland.

Carey, B. (2007). Do you believe in magic? *New York Times,* January 23.

Conrad, K. (1958). *Die beginnende schizophrenie. Versuch einer gestaltanalyse des wahns.* Stuttgart: Thieme. Discussed in S. Banbury and S. Tremblay, eds. (2004). *A cognitive approach to situation awareness: Theory and application.* Aldershot, UK: Ashgate.

Druckman, D., and J. A. Swets, eds. (1988). *Enhancing human performance: Issues, theories, and techniques.* Washington, DC: National Academy Press.

Gazzaniga, M. S. (2005). *The ethical brain.* New York: Dana Press.

Gmelch, G. (1992). Superstition and ritual in American baseball. *Elysian Fields Quarterly* 11(3): 25–36.

Hood, B. (2006). The intuitive magician: Why belief in the supernatural persists. *Cerebrum,* July 1. http://www.dana.org/news/cerebrum/detail.aspx?id=114.

Jahoda, G. (1974). *The psychology of superstition.* New York: Jason Aronson.

Lindeman, M., and K. Aarnio. (2006). Superstitious, magical, and paranormal beliefs: An integrative model. *Journal of Research in Personality* 41(4): 731–744.

Lindeman, M., and M. Saher. (2007). Vitalism, purpose and superstition. *British Journal of Psychology* 98(1): 33–44.

Ono, K. (1987). Superstitious behavior in humans. *Journal of the Experimental Analysis of Behavior* 47(3): 261–271.

————. (1997). Response stereotypy in humans maintained by response-contingent events. *Japanese Psychological Research* 39(4): 277–290.

Porter, D. (2007). Larsen, Berra see perfect game broadcast. Associated Press, February 23.

Pronin, E., D. M. Wegner, K. McCarthy, and S. Rodriguez. (2006). Everyday magical powers: The role of apparent mental causation in the overestimation of personal influence. *Journal of Personality and Social Psychology* 91(2): 218–231.

Rozin, P., L. Millman and C. Nemeroff. (1986). Operation of the laws of sympathy magic in disgust and other domains. Journal of Personality and Social Psychology 50: 703–712.

Skinner, B. F. (1947). "Superstition" in the pigeon. *Journal of Experimental Psychology* 38: 168–172.

Stone, L. (2005). The art of baseball: A tradition of superstition. *Seattle Times*, September 26.

Vyse, S. A. (2000). *Believing in magic: The psychology of superstition.* New York: Oxford University Press.

Wagner, G. A. and E. K. Morris. (1987). "Superstitious" behavior in children. *The Psychological Record* 37:471–488.

CHAPTER 5

Barnes, M. (1989). Dock Ellis is ready to shed flaky image to be an agent. United Press International, June 20.

Beilock, S. L., and T. H. Carr. (2001). On the fragility of skilled performance: What governs choking under pressure? *Journal of Experimental Psychology: General* 130(4): 701–725.

Beiner, J. M., P. Jokl, J. Cholewicki, and M. M. Panjabi. (1999). The effect of anabolic steroids and corticosteroids on healing of muscle contusion injury. *American Journal of Sports Medicine* 27(1): 2–9.

Bloom, B. M. (2003). Many players applaud testing. *MLB.com,* November 14. http://www.mlb.com/news/article.jsp?ymd=20031114&content_id=604197&vkey=news_mlb&fext=.jsp&c_id=mlb (accessed August 13, 2007).

Bouton, J. (1970). *Ball four: My life and hard times throwing the knuckleball in the big leagues.* New York: World Publishing.

de Wit, H., J. L. Enggasser, and J. B. Richards. (2002). Acute administration of *d*-amphetamine decreases impulsivity in healthy volunteers. *Neuropsychopharmacology* 27: 813–825.

Eagle, D. M., M. R. Tufft, H. L. Goodchild, and T. W. Robbins. (2007). Differential effects of modafinil and methylphenidate on stop-signal reaction time task performance in the rat, and interactions with the dopamine receptor antagonist *cis*-flupenthixol. *Psychopharmacology* 192(2): 193–206.

Freeman, M., and B. Olney. (2003). New drug tests in baseball stir debate among players. *New York Times,* April 22.

Hienz, R. D., D. J. Spear, and D. A. Bowers. (1994). Effects of cocaine on simple reaction times and sensory thresholds in baboons. *Journal of the Experimental Analysis of Behavior* 61(2): 231–246.

O'Toole, A. (2003). *The best man plays: Major league baseball and the black athlete, 1901–2002.* Jefferson, NC: McFarland.

Rasch, P. J., W. R. Pierson, and M. L. Brubaker. (1960). The effect of amphetamine sulfate and meprobamate on reaction time and movement time. *European Journal of Applied Physiology* 18(3): 280–284.

Shackman, A. J., I. Sarinopoulos, J. S. Maxwell, D. A. Pizzagalli, A. Lavric, and R. J. Davidson. (2006). Anxiety selectively disrupts visuospatial working memory. *Emotion* 6(1): 40–61.

Tedeschi, G., P. R. M. Bittencourt, A. T. Smith, and A. Richens. (1983). Effect of amphetamine on saccadic and smooth pursuit eye movements. *Psychopharmacology* 79(2–3): 190–192.

Turner, D. C., T. W. Robbins, L. Clark, A. R. Aron, J. Dowson, and B. J. Sahakian. (2003). Cognitive enhancing effects of modafinil in healthy volunteers. *Psychopharmacology* 165(3): 260–269.

World Anti-Doping Agency. (2003). *World anti-doping code.* Montreal: World Anti-Doping Agency.

———. (2007). 2007 budget summary. http://www.wada-ama.org/rtecontent/document/2007_Budget_Expenditures.pdf.

CHAPTER 6

Annett, M. (1970). A classification of hand preference by association analysis. *British Journal of Psychology* 61: 303–321.

Branch, C., B. Milner, and T. Rasmussen. (1964). Intracarotid sodium amytal for the lateralization of cerebral speech dominance: Observations in 123 patients. *Journal of Neurosurgery* 21: 399–405.

Broca, P. (1865). Sur la faculté du language articulé. Bulletins et Mémoires de la Société d'Anthropologie de Paris 6: 337–393.

Bryden, M. P. (1982). *Laterality: Functional asymmetry in the intact brain.* New York: Academic Press.

Foundas, A. L., K. Hong, C. M. Leonard, and K. M. Heilman. (1998). Hand preference and magnetic resonance imaging asymmetries of the central sulcus. *Neuropsychiatry, Neuropsychology, and Behavioral Neurology* 11(2): 65–71.

Foundas, A. L., C. M. Leonard, R. Gilmore, E. Fennell, and K. M. Heilman. (1994). Planum temporale asymmetry and language dominance. *Neuropsychologia* 32(10): 1225–1231.

Geschwind, N., and W. Levitsky. (1968). Human brain: Left-right asymmetries in temporal speech region. *Science* 161: 186–187.

Gilbert, A. N., and C. J. Wisocki. (1992). Hand preference and age in the United States. *Neuropsychologia* 30: 601–608.

Graff-Radford, J., G. P. Crucian, and K. M. Heilman. (2006). The right arm likes to be close. *Cortex* 42(5): 699–704.

Grondin, S., M. Trottier, and C. Houle. (1994). Préférences manuelle et latérale et style de jeu au hockey sur glace [Manual and lateral preferences and playing style in ice hockey]. *Revue des Sciences et Techniques des Activités Physiques et Sportives* 35: 65–75.

Healey, J. M., J. Liederman, and N. Geschwind. (1986). Handedness is not a unidimensional trait. *Cortex* 22(1): 33–53.

Heilman, K. M., A. Chatterjee, and L. C. Doty. (1995). Hemispheric asymmetries of near-far spatial attention. *Neuropsychology* 9(1): 58–61.

Heilman, K. M., J. M. Coyle, E. F. Gonyea, and N. Geschwind. (1973). Apraxia and agraphia in a left-hander. *Brain* 96(1): 21–28.

Heilman, K. M., and L. J. G. Rothi. (2003). Apraxia. In *Clinical neuropsychology,* 4th ed., ed. K. M. Heilman and E. Valenstein, 215–235. Oxford: Oxford University Press.

Hore, J., S. Watts, D. Tweed, and B. Miller. (1996). Overarm throws with the nondominant arm: Kinematics of accuracy. *Journal of Neurophysiology* 76(6): 3693–3704.

Kuypers, H. G. J. M. (1962). Corticospinal connections: Postnatal development in the rhesus monkey. *Science* 138: 678–680.

Liepmann, H. (1920). Apraxia. *Ergebnisse der Gesamten Medizin* 1: 516–543.

Liepmann, H., and O. Maas. (1907). Fall von linksseitiger Agraphie und Apraxie bei rechtsseitiger Lähmung. *Journal für Psychologie und Neurologie* 10: 214–227.

Masure, M. C., and A. L. Benton. (1983). Visuospatial performance in left-handed patients with unilateral brain lesions. *Neuropsychologia* 21(2): 179–181.

McLean, J. M., and F. M. Ciurczak. (1982). Bimanual dexterity in major league baseball players: A statistical study. *New England Journal of Medicine* 307(20): 1278–1279.

McManus, I. C., C. Porac, M. P. Bryden, and R. Boucher. (1999). Eye-dominance, writing hand, and throwing hand. *Laterality* 4(2): 173–192.

Mühlau, M., J. Hermsdörfer, G. Goldenberg, A. M. Wohlschläger, F. Castrop, R. Stahl, M. Röttinger, P. Erhard, B. Haslinger, A. O. Ceballos-Baumann, B. Conrad, and H. Boecker. (2005). Left inferior parietal dominance in gesture imitation: An fMRI study. *Neuropsychologia* 43(7): 1086–1098.

Porac, C., and S. Coren. (1981). *Lateral preferences and human behavior.* New York: Springer-Verlag.

Portal, J. M., and P. E. Romano. (1988). Patterns of eye-hand dominance in baseball players. *New England Journal of Medicine* 319: 655–656.

Rao, S. M., P. A. Bandettini, J. R. Binder, J. A. Bobholz, T. A. Hammeke, E. A. Stein, and J. S. Hyde. (1996). Relationship between finger movement rate and functional magnetic resonance signal change in human primary motor cortex. *Journal of Cerebal Blood Flow and Metabolism* 16(6): 1250–1254.

Rapcsak, S. Z., L. J. Gonzalez Rothi, and K. M. Heilman. (1987). Apraxia in a patient with atypical cerebral dominance. *Brain and Cognition* 6(4): 450–463.

Rasmussen, T. and B. Milner. (1975). Clinical and surgical studies of the cerebral speech areas in man. In: Zülch, K.J., O. Creutzfeldt, and G.C. Galbraith (editors). Cerebral localization. Berlin: Springer-Verlag. pp. 238–257.

Roth, H. L., A. N. Lora, and K. M. Heilman. (2002). Effects of monocular viewing and eye dominance on spatial attention. *Brain* 125: 2023–2035.

Taylor, H. G., and K. M. Heilman. (1980). Left-hemisphere motor dominance in right handers. *Cortex* 16(4): 587–603.

Valenstein, E., and K. M. Heilman. (1979). Apraxic agraphia with neglect-induced paragraphia. *Archives of Neurology* 36(8): 506–508.

Verfaellie, M., and K. M. Heilman. (1990). Hemispheric asymmetries in attentional control: Implications for hand preference in sensorimotor tasks. *Brain and Cognition* 14(1): 70–80.

Watson, R. T., and K. M. Heilman. (1983). Callosal apraxia. *Brain* 106: 391–403.

CHAPTER 7

Azari, N. P., J. Missimer, and R. J. Seitz. (2005). Religious experience and emotion: Evidence for distinctive cognitive neural patterns. *International Journal for the Psychology of Religion* 15: 263–281.

Azari, N. P., J. Nickel, G. Wunderlich, M. Niedeggen, H. Hefter, L. Tellmann, H. Herzog, P. Stoerig, D. Birnbacher, and R. J. Seitz. (2001). Neural correlates of religious experience. *European Journal of Neuroscience* 13: 1649–1652.

Bernhardt, P. C., J. M. Dabbs Jr., J. A. Fielden, and D. C. Lutter. (1998). Testosterone changes during vicarious experiences of winning and losing among fans at sporting events. *Physiology and Behavior* 65: 59–62.

Blood, A. J., and R. J. Zatorre. (2001). Intensely pleasurable responses to music correlate with activity in brain regions implicated in reward and emotion. *Proceedings of the National Academy of Sciences* 98: 11818–11823.

Borg, J., B. Andrée, H. Soderstrom, and L. Farde. (2003). The serotonin system and spiritual experiences. *American Journal of Psychiatry* 160: 1965–1969.

Breiter, H. C., I. Aharon, D. Kahneman, A. Dale, and P. Shizgal. (2001). Functional imaging of neural responses to expectancy and experience of monetary gains and losses. *Neuron* 30: 619–639.

Cohen, M. X., J. Young, J. M. Baek, C. Kessler, and C. Ranganath. (2005). Individual differences in extraversion and dopamine genetics predict neural reward responses. *Cognitive Brain Research* 25: 851–861.

God on the brain. (2003). *Horizon,* BBC TV & Radio, April 17.

Holland, P. C., and M. Gallagher. (2004). Amygdala-frontal interactions and reward expectancy. *Current Opinion in Neurobiology* 14: 148–155.

Horgan, J. (2006). The God experiments: Five researchers take science where it's never gone before. *Discover,* November 11. http://discovermagazine.com/2006/dec/god-experiments.

Kringelbach, M. L. (2005). The human orbitofrontal cortex: Linking reward to hedonic experience. *Nature Reviews Neuroscience* 6: 691–702.

Kübler-Ross, E. [1969] (1997). *On death and dying.* Repr. New York: Touchstone.

Najib, A., J. P. Lorberbaum, S. Kose, D. E. Bohning, and M. S. George. (2004). Regional brain activity in women grieving a romantic relationship breakup. *American Journal of Psychiatry* 161: 2245–2256.

Olds, J., and P. Milner. (1954). Positive reinforcement produced by electrical stimulation of septal area and other regions of rat brain. *Journal of Comparative and Physiological Psychology* 47: 419–427.

Senor, T. D. (2004). Should Cubs fans be committed? What bleacher bums have to tell us about the nature of faith. In *Baseball and philosophy: Thinking outside the batter's box,* ed. E. Bronson, 37–55. Chicago: Open Court Press.

Wicker, B., C. Keysers, J. Plailly, J. P. Royet, V. Gallese, and G. Rizzolatti. (2003). Both of us disgusted in my insula: The common neural basis of seeing and feeling disgust. *Neuron* 40: 655–664.

CONTRIBUTORS

JORDAN GRAFMAN, PH.D., is a senior investigator at the National Institute for Neurological Disorders and Stroke, part of the National Institutes of Health. He has served as chief of the Cognitive Neuroscience Section of NINDS since 1989. He is an elected Fellow of the American Psychological Association and has received both the Defense Meritorious Service Award for his studies of brain-injured Vietnam veterans and the National Institutes of Health Award of Merit. He was born and raised in the City of Chicago.

SCOTT GRAFTON, M.D., is a neurologist with expertise in brain imaging and human motor systems. He directs the imaging center at the University of California at Santa Barbara and is the author of more than 125 publications on skill learning, action representation, and understanding action in other people. His work has helped reveal how patients with disorders such as Parkinson's disease or stroke reorganize their motor systems to accomplish goal-directed behavior.

JOHN MILTON, M.D., PH.D., F.R.C.P.C., is the William R. Kenan Jr. Chair of Computational Neuroscience at the Claremont Colleges in California and a Fellow of the American Physical Society. His current research interests focus on the development of expert motor skills by the human nervous system. He has written more than 100 articles and three books.

ANA SOLODKIN, PH.D., is a research associate, assistant professor in the Department of Neurology at the University of Chicago. Her active and long-term research has focused on the relationship between basic neurobiology and cognitive neurology, with an emphasis on degenerative disorders (cerebellar ataxias and Alzheimer's disease) and motor recovery from stroke.

STEVEN L. SMALL, PH.D., M.D., is professor of neurology and psychology at the University of Chicago and a member of the Graduate Committees on Neurobiology and Computational Neuroscience. His work focuses on the cognitive and computational neurobiology of language and motor function, both in the normally functioning state and after neurological injury.

TOM VALEO is a freelance writer in St. Petersburg, Florida, who writes frequently about neurology, psychology, and aging.

LINDSAY BEYERSTEIN is an investigative journalist in New York City. Her print reporting has appeared in *Salon*, *Slate*, *New York Press*, *AlterNet*, and other publications.

BENNETT FODDY, PH.D., holds the Harold T. Shapiro Fellowship in Bioethics at Princeton University's Center for Human Values. He is the author of numerous articles about human enhancement and sport, including "Can Addicted People Consent to the Prescription of their Drug?" in *Bioethics* and "The Ethics of Performance Enhancement in Sport: Drugs and Gene Doping" in *Principles of Health Care Ethics*.

KENNETH M. HEILMAN, M.D., is the James E. Rooks Jr. Distinguished Professor of Neurology & Health Psychology at the University of Florida College of Medicine and neurology chief at the North Florida–South Georgia Veterans Affairs Health System in Gainesville, Florida.

KELLI WHITLOCK BURTON has covered science and medicine for seventeen years as a staff reporter and a freelance writer. She currently lives near Columbus, Ohio, and writes for *Science*, the *Boston Globe*, *ScienceNOW*, and several Dana Press publications.

HILLARY R. RODMAN, PH.D., is an associate professor of psychology at Emory University, where she teaches a course called Science and Myth of Baseball. She studies the brain systems that govern high-level visual abilities such as object recognition and the awareness of stimuli.

INDEX

OTHER DANA PRESS BOOKS AND PERIODICALS

www.dana.org/books/press

BOOKS FOR GENERAL READERS
BRAIN AND MIND:

THE NEUROSCIENCE OF FAIR PLAY: *Why We (Usually) Follow the Golden Rule*

Donald W. Pfaff, Ph.D.

Foreword by Edward O. Wilson

Pfaff explains how specific brain circuits cause us to consider an action toward another as if it were going to happen to us, prompting us to treat others as we wish to be treated ourselves. Pfaff solves the mystery of our universal ethical precepts, presenting a rock-solid hypothesis of why humans across time and geography have such similar notions of good and bad, right and wrong. 10 halftone illustrations.

Cloth, 300 pp. • $23.95

ISBN-13: 978-1-932594-27-0

BEST OF THE BRAIN FROM SCIENTIFIC AMERICAN: *Mind, Matter, and Tomorrow's Brain*

Floyd E. Bloom, M.D., Editor

Top neuroscientist Floyd E. Bloom has selected the most fascinating brain-related articles from *Scientific American* and *Scientific American Mind* since 1999 in this collection. Divided into three sections—Mind, Matter, and Tomorrow's Brain—this compilation offers the latest information from the front lines of brain research. 30 full-color illustrations.

Cloth, 261 pp. • $25.00

ISBN-13: 978-1-932594-22-5

CEREBRUM 2007: *Emerging Ideas in Brain Science*
Cynthia A. Read, Editor
Foreword by Bruce McEwen, Ph.D.

Prominent scientists and other thinkers explain, applaud, and protest new ideas arising from discoveries about the brain in this first yearly anthology from *Cerebrum's* Web journal for inquisitive general readers. 10 black-and-white illustrations.

Paper 243 pp. • $14.95

ISBN-13: 978-1-932594-24-9

MIND WARS: *Brain Research and National Defense*
Jonathan Moreno, Ph.D.

A leading ethicist examines national security agencies' work on defense applications of brain science, and the ethical issues to consider.

Cloth 210 pp. • $23.95

ISBN-13: 978-1-932594-16-4

THE DANA GUIDE TO BRAIN HEALTH: *A Practical Family Reference from Medical Experts (with CD-ROM)*
Floyd E. Bloom, M.D., M. Flint Beal, M.D., and
David J. Kupfer, M.D., Editors
Foreword by William Safire

The only complete, authoritative family-friendly guide to the brain's development, health, and disorders. *The Dana Guide to Brain Health* offers ready reference to our latest understanding of brain diseases as well as information to help you participate in your family's care. 16 full-color illustrations and more than 200 black-and-white drawings.

Paper (with CD-ROM) 733 pp. • $25.00

ISBN-13: 978-1-932594-10-2

THE CREATING BRAIN: *The Neuroscience of Genius*
Nancy C. Andreasen, M.D., Ph.D.

A noted psychiatrist and bestselling author explores how the brain achieves creative breakthroughs, including questions such as how creative people are different and the difference between genius and intelligence. She also describes how to develop our creative capacity. 33 illustrations/photos.

Cloth 197 pp. • $23.95

ISBN-13: 978-1-932594-07-2

THE ETHICAL BRAIN
Michael S. Gazzaniga, Ph.D.

Explores how the lessons of neuroscience help resolve today's ethical dilemmas, ranging from when life begins to free will and criminal responsibility. The author, a pioneer in cognitive neuroscience, is a member of the President's Council on Bioethics.

Cloth 201 pp.1-932594-01-9 • $25.00

A GOOD START IN LIFE: *Understanding Your Child's Brain and Behavior from Birth to Age 6*
Norbert Herschkowitz, M.D., and Elinore Chapman Herschkowitz

The authors show how brain development shapes a child's personality and behavior, discussing appropriate rule-setting, the child's moral sense, temperament, language, playing, aggression, impulse control, and empathy. 13 illustrations.

Cloth 283 pp. 0-309-07639-0 • $22.95
Paper (Updated with new material) 312 pp. 0-9723830-5-0 • $13.95

BACK FROM THE BRINK: *How Crises Spur Doctors to New Discoveries about the Brain*
Edward J. Sylvester

In two academic medical centers, Columbia's New York Presbyterian and Johns Hopkins Medical Institutions, a new breed of doctor, the neurointensivist, saves patients with life-threatening brain injuries. 16 illustrations/photos.

Cloth 296 pp. 0-9723830-4-2 • $25.00

THE BARD ON THE BRAIN: *Understanding the Mind Through the Art of Shakespeare and the Science of Brain Imaging*
Paul Matthews, M.D., and Jeffrey McQuain, Ph.D.
Foreword by Diane Ackerman

Explores the beauty and mystery of the human mind and the workings of the brain, following the path the Bard pointed out in 35 of the most famous speeches from his plays. 100 illustrations.

Cloth 248 pp. 0-9723830-2-6 • $35.00

STRIKING BACK AT STROKE: *A Doctor-Patient Journal*
Cleo Hutton and Louis R. Caplan, M.D.

A personal account with medical guidance from a leading neurologist for anyone enduring the changes that a stroke can bring to a life, a family, and a sense of self. 15 illustrations.

Cloth 240 pp. 0-9723830-1-8 • $27.00

UNDERSTANDING DEPRESSION:
What We Know and What You Can Do About It
J. Raymond DePaulo Jr., M.D., and Leslie Alan Horvitz.
Foreword by Kay Redfield Jamison, Ph.D.

What depression is, who gets it and why, what happens in the brain, troubles that come with the illness, and the treatments that work.

Cloth 304 pp. 0-471-39552-8 • $24.95

Paper 296 pp. 0-471-43030-7 • $14.95

KEEP YOUR BRAIN YOUNG: *The Complete Guide to Physical and Emotional Health and Longevity*
Guy McKhann, M.D., and Marilyn Albert, Ph.D.

Every aspect of aging and the brain: changes in memory, nutrition, mood, sleep, and sex, as well as the later problems in alcohol use, vision, hearing, movement, and balance.

Cloth 304 pp. 0-471-40792-5 • $24.95

Paper 304 pp. 0-471-43028-5 • $15.95

THE END OF STRESS AS WE KNOW IT
Bruce McEwen, Ph.D., with Elizabeth Norton Lasley
Foreword by Robert Sapolsky

How brain and body work under stress and how it is possible to avoid its debilitating effects.

Cloth 239 pp. 0-309-07640-4 • $27.95

Paper 262 pp. 0-309-09121-7 • $19.95

IN SEARCH OF THE LOST CORD: *Solving the Mystery*
of Spinal Cord Regeneration
Luba Vikhanski

The story of the scientists and science involved in the international scientific race to find ways to repair the damaged spinal cord and restore movement. 21 photos; 12 illustrations.

Cloth 269 pp. 0-309-07437-1 • $27.95

THE SECRET LIFE OF THE BRAIN
Richard Restak, M.D.
Foreword by David Grubin

Companion book to the PBS series of the same name, exploring recent discoveries about the brain from infancy through old age.

Cloth 201 pp. 0-309-07435-5 • $35.00

THE LONGEVITY STRATEGY: *How to Live to 100*
Using the Brain-Body Connection
David Mahoney and Richard Restak, M.D.
Foreword by William Safire

Advice on the brain and aging well.

Cloth 250 pp. 0-471-24867-3 • $22.95
Paper 272 pp. 0-471-32794-8 • $14.95

STATES OF MIND: *New Discoveries about*
How Our Brains Make Us Who We Are
Roberta Conlan, Editor

Adapted from the Dana/Smithsonian Associates lecture series by eight of the country's top brain scientists, including the 2000 Nobel laureate in medicine, Eric Kandel.

Cloth 214 pp. 0-471-29963-4 • $24.95
Paper 224 pp. 0-471-39973-6 • $18.95

BEYOND THERAPY: *Biotechnology and the Pursuit of Happiness.*

A Report of the President's Council on Bioethics

Special Foreword by Leon R. Kass, M.D., Chairman.

Introduction by William Safire

Can biotechnology satisfy human desires for better children, superior performance, ageless bodies, and happy souls? This report says these possibilities present us with profound ethical challenges and choices. Includes dissenting commentary by scientist members of the Council.

Paper 376 pp. 1-932594-05-1 • $10.95

NEUROETHICS: *Mapping the Field. Conference Proceedings.*

Steven J. Marcus, Editor

Proceedings of the landmark 2002 conference organized by Stanford University and the University of California, San Francisco, and sponsored by The Dana Foundation, at which more than 150 neuroscientists, bioethicists, psychiatrists and psychologists, philosophers, and professors of law and public policy debated the ethical implications of neuroscience research findings. 50 illustrations.

Paper 367 pp. 0-9723830-0-X • $10.95

IMMUNOLOGY:

RESISTANCE: *The Human Struggle Against Infection*

Norbert Gualde, M.D., translated by Steven Rendall

Traces the histories of epidemics and the emergence or re-emergence of diseases, illustrating how new global strategies and research of the body's own weapons of immunity can work together to fight tomorrow's inevitable infectious outbreaks.

Cloth 219 pp. • $25.00

ISBN-13: 978-1-932594-00-3

FATAL SEQUENCE: *The Killer Within*
Kevin J. Tracey, M.D.

An easily understood account of the spiral of sepsis, a sometimes fatal crisis that most often affects patients fighting off nonfatal illnesses or injury. Tracey puts the scientific and medical story of sepsis in the context of his battle to save a burned baby, a sensitive telling of cutting-edge science.

Cloth 225 pp. 1-932594-06-X • $23.95

Paper 225 pp. 1-932594-09-4 • $12.95

ARTS EDUCATION

A WELL-TEMPERED MIND: *Using Music to Help Children Listen and Learn*
Peter Perret and Janet Fox
Foreword by Maya Angelou

Five musicians enter elementary school classrooms, helping children learn about music and contributing to both higher enthusiasm and improved academic performance. This charming story gives us a taste of things to come in one of the newest areas of brain research: the effect of music on the brain. 12 illustrations.

Cloth 231 pp. 1-932594-03-5 • $22.95

Paper 231 pp. 1-932594-08-6 • $12.00

FREE EDUCATIONAL BOOKS

(Information about ordering and downloadable PDFs are available at *www.dana.org.*)

PARTNERING ARTS EDUCATION: *A Working Model from ArtsConnection*

This publication describes how classroom teachers and artists learned to form partnerships as they built successful residencies in schools. *Partnering Arts Education* provides insight and concrete steps in the ArtsConnection model. 55 pp.

ACTS OF ACHIEVEMENT: *The Role of*
Performing Arts Centers in Education.

Profiles of more than 60 programs, plus eight extended case studies, from urban and rural communities across the United States, illustrating different approaches to performing arts education programs in school settings. Black-and-white photos throughout. 164 pp.

PLANNING AN ARTS-CENTERED SCHOOL: *A Handbook*

A practical guide for those interested in creating, maintaining, or upgrading arts-centered schools. Includes curriculum and development, governance, funding, assessment, and community participation. Black-and-white photos throughout. 164 pp.

THE DANA SOURCEBOOK OF BRAIN SCIENCE: *Resources for*
Teachers and Students, Fourth Edition

A basic introduction to brain science, its history, current understanding of the brain, new developments, and future directions. 16 color photos; 29 black-and-white photos; 26 black-and- white illustrations. 160 pp.

THE DANA SOURCEBOOK OF IMMUNOLOGY:
Resources for Secondary and Post-Secondary Teachers and Students

An introduction to how the immune system protects us, what happens when it breaks down, the diseases that threaten it, and the unique relationship between the immune system and the brain. 5 color photos; 36 black-and-white photos; 11 black-and-white illustrations. 116 pp. ISSN: 1558-6758

PERIODICALS

Dana Press also offers several periodicals dealing with arts education, immunology, and brain science. These periodicals are available free to subscribers by mail. Please visit *www.dana.org*.